HORMONE RECEPTORS

ADVANCES IN EXPERIMENTAL MEDICINE AND BIOLOGY

HORMONE RECEPTORS

Edited by

David M. Klachko
Leonard R. Forte
and
John M. Franz
University of Missouri - Columbia

SPRINGER SCIENCE+BUSINESS MEDIA, LLC

Library of Congress Cataloging in Publication Data

Midwest Conference on Endocrinology and Metabolism, 11th, University of Missouri—
Columbia, 1975.
   Hormone receptors.
   (Advances in Experimental Medicine and Biology; v. 96)
   Includes index.
   1. Hormone receptors—Congresses. I. Klachko, David M. II. Forte, Leonard R. III. Franz,
John M. IV. Title. [DNLM: 1. Receptors, Hormone—Congresses. W3 MI307E 1975h/WK102
M629 1975h]
QP188.5.H67M5 1975   599'.01'927   77-25856
ISBN 978-1-4757-0724-3   ISBN 978-1-4757-0722-9 (eBook)
DOI 10.1007/978-1-4757-0722-9

Proceedings of the Eleventh Midwest Conference on Endocrinology and Metabolism held at
the University of Missouri, Columbia, Missouri, October 2–3, 1975 and sponsored by:

   University of Missouri-Columbia
      College of Agriculture
      College of Veterinary Medicine
      Dalton Research Center
      Department of Biochemistry
      Department of Medicine
      Department of Pharmacology
      Department of Physiology
      Department of Veterinary Pathology
      Division of Biological Sciences
      Graduate School
      School of Medicine
      Sinclair Comparative Med. Res. Farm
   American Chemical Society - UMC Chapter
   Ayerst Company
   Ciba-Geigy Corporation
   Harry S. Truman Memorial Veterans Hospital
   Merck, Sharp and Dohme
   G.D. Searle and Company
   The Upjohn Company

© 1978 Springer Science+Business Media New York
Originally published by Plenum Press, New York in 1978

CONFERENCE CHAIRMAN

DAVID M. KLACHKO, M.D., Associate Professor of Medicine, University of Missouri-Columbia

PLANNING COMMITTEE

CONSTANTINE S. ANAST, M.D., Professor of Child Health, University of Missouri-Columbia

RALPH R. ANDERSON, Ph.D., Associate Professor of Dairy Husbandry, University of Missouri-Columbia

JOHN D. DAVID, Ph.D., Assistant Professor of Biological Sciences, University of Missouri-Columbia

HORST-DIETER DELLMANN, Dr. med. vet., Ph.D., Professor of Veterinary Anatomy-Physiology, University of Missouri-Columbia

LEONARD R. FORTE, Ph.D., Associate Professor of Pharmacology, University of Missouri-Columbia

JOHN M. FRANZ, Ph.D., Associate Professor of Biochemistry, University of Missouri-Columbia

JAMES A. GREEN, Ph.D., Professor of Anatomy, University of Missouri-Columbia

LAURENCE W. HEDLUND, Ph.D., Assistant Professor of Dairy Husbandry, University of Missouri-Columbia

MURRAY HEIMBERG, Ph.D., M.D., Professor and Chairman, Department of Pharmacology; Professor of Medicine, University of Missouri-Columbia

J. ALAN JOHNSON, Ph.D., Assistant Professor of Physiology, University of Missouri-Columbia

HAROLD LAMB, Conference Coordinator, Conferences and Short Courses, University Extension Division, University of Missouri-Columbia

WARREN L. ZAHLER, Ph.D., Assistant Professor of Biochemistry, University of Missouri-Columbia

SPEAKERS

ROBERT N. BRADY, Ph.D., Assistant Professor of Biochemistry, Vanderbilt University, Nashville, Tennessee

LESLIE J. DEGROOT, M.D., Professor of Medicine, University of Chicago and Pritzker School of Medicine, Chicago, Illinois

PHILIP FEIGELSON, Ph.D., Professor of Biochemistry, Institute of Cancer Research, College of Physicians and Surgeons of Columbia University, New York, New York

OSCAR M. HECHTER, Ph.D., Chairman and Nathan Smith Davis Professor of Physiology, Northwestern University Medical School, Chicago, Illinois

ROBERT J. LEFKOWITZ, M.D., Associate Professor of Medicine, Assistant Professor of Biochemistry, Duke University Medical Center, Durham, North Carolina

ARLAN L. ROSENBLOOM, M.D., Professor of Pediatrics, University of Florida, Gainesville, Florida

WILLIAM T. SCHRADER, Ph.D., Assistant Professor of Cell Biology, Baylor College of Medicine, Houston, Texas

MODERATORS

BENEDICT J. CAMPBELL, Ph.D., Professor and Chairman, Department of Biochemistry, University of Missouri-Columbia

LEONARD R. FORTE, Ph.D., Associate Professor of Pharmacology, University of Missouri-Columbia

MURRAY HEIMBERG, Ph.D., M.D., Professor and Chairman, Department of Pharmacology; Professor of Medicine, University of Missouri-Columbia

EDWARD SIEGEL, Ph.D., Professor of Medicine and Radiology, University of Missouri-Columbia

DISCUSSANTS

BARNAWELL, E.B., School of Life Sciences, University of Nebraska, Lincoln, Nebraska

BLACK, A.C. Jr., Department of Anatomy, University of Iowa, Iowa City, Iowa

BURNS, T.W., Department of Medicine, University of Missouri-Columbia

CAMPBELL, B.J., Department of Biochemistry, University of Missouri-Columbia

FORTE, L.R., Department of Pharmacology, University of Missouri-Columbia

FRANZ, J.M., Department of Biochemistry, University of Missouri-Columbia

FREED, W.J., Department of Human Development and Family Life, University of Kansas, Lawrence, Kansas

HAGEN, G.A., Medical Service, Veterans Administration Hospital, St. Louis, Missouri

HEIMBERG, M., Department of Pharmacology, University of Missouri-Columbia

KLACHKO, D.M., Department of Medicine, University of Missouri-Columbia

KORNEL, L., Steroid Unit, Department of Medicine, Rush-Presbyterian-St. Luke's Medical Center, Chicago, Illinois

LATA, G.F., Department of Biochemistry, University of Iowa, Iowa City, Iowa

MORGAN, D.W., Department of Biochemistry, University of Missouri-Columbia

PRAHLAD, K.V., Department of Biological Sciences, Northern Illinois University, DeKalb, Illinois

SIEGEL, E., Departments of Medicine and Radiology, University of Missouri-Columbia

SUN, A., Sinclair Research Farm, Columbia, Missouri

TRIANO, J.J., Logan College of Chiropractic, Chesterfield, Missouri

Preface

The Eleventh Midwest Conference on Endocrinology and Metabolism in September 1975 brought together a number of leading investigators in the areas of steroid, peptide, acetylcholine, and catecholamine hormone receptor studies. This book is based upon the reports of investigations into hormone receptor biochemistry and physiology presented at the Conference as well as on the ensuing discussions. However, many of the manuscripts were written after the Conference. Because of this, the reader will find that some literature references and results of investigations are more up-to-date than the Conference date would suggest.

Perusal of this and previous volumes will attest to the high quality of this annual conference, due primarily to the efforts of the Planning Committee. We also acknowledge the superb efforts of the staff of Conferences and Short Courses for their assistance in organizing the Conference, and Mrs. Linda Bennett for expert secretarial assistance in the typing of the book. Last, but certainly not least, we express our appreciation to the various organizations that provided the necessary financial assistance.

Leonard R. Forte
John M. Franz
David M. Klachko

Preface

Contents

THE RECEPTOR CONCEPT: PREJUDICE, PREDICTION, AND PARADOX*

Oscar Hechter

Department of Physiology
Northwestern University Medical School
303 E. Chicago Avenue
Chicago, IL 60611

INTRODUCTION

This is a time of "great expectations" in the field of hormone and neurotransmitter action. Recent advances in our understanding of receptors have been so dramatic that we appear to be at the threshold of finally resolving the molecular nature of cellular receptors. The nature of these receptors is an important issue in biology which transcends endocrinology and neural transmission; it concerns the cardinal problem in the broad area of intercellular and intracellular communication. The once "elusive" receptors for hormones and neurotransmitters, long postulated to be the primary functional units for initiation of biological action, now appear to be "real" molecules. Specific macromolecular binding units for certain hormones and transmitters, with kinetic and specificity characteristics expected for a receptor have been reported. They can be isolated and manipulated. In several cases these receptors, derived either from the "cytosol" or solubilized from plasma membranes have been isolated in pure form. It is widely accepted that if we now follow the same strategy so successfully employed by the enzymologists (first isolate, then proceed to chemical characterization and determination of subunit sequences, conformational analysis, finally X-ray analysis) that the intimate molecular details of receptor structure and function will be clarified.

If this is a period of great excitement and enthusiasm, it is also a period of great competition. Several major research groups

*The studies described have been aided by grants from the Rockefeller Foundation and NIH Grant PO 1-HD-06273.

working on one receptor or another, all using essentially a similar strategy, are actively competing for the next "key" finding and
the prizes (Nobel and otherwise) which reward major achievements
in biomedical research. The competing research teams share the
feeling that the basic concepts and most of the technology necessary to finish the job are already at hand. The constraints to
further progress and eventual success are perceived to be those
operative at the fiscal level; the problem is to obtain major
funding at a period in history where money for basic sciences is
in very short supply, and there are a multiplicity of competing
demands (in and out of science).

Do these expectations, rarely expressed explicitly but widely
held privately, correspond to reality? Granted that dramatic advances have, indeed, been made, and that further progress can be
clearly envisaged, are we really at the threshold of solving the
receptor problem? Does it follow that once the molecular details
of receptor structure are clarified one by one, that the causative
basis of receptor function will necessarily become clear and obvious? There is no such inevitability. There may well be com-
plexities of such a nature that the receptor problem, in all its
dimensions, will not be solved by following previous "road maps."
The latter statement implies that we may need new fundamental concepts (as well as new techniques) if we are to resolve the receptor
problem. One thesis of this presentation is that our concepts of
receptors are incomplete until we can explain how receptors function to "initiate" physiological action. This involves a precise
description of how the "occupied" receptor is "coupled" (both in
cybernetic and energetic terms) to "secondary" functional units.
Let us remember that despite spectacular achievements in enzymol-
ogy and molecular structure, the precise mechanisms and principles
underlying energy coupling in biological systems remain a subject
of great controversy and debate. The "coupling problem" in hormone action is not necessarily simpler than the problem of energy
coupling in oxidative phosphorylation.

Having introduced a cautionary note in provocative fashion,
let me remind you of the historical process by which a dynamic
science advances, once it has achieved maturity. Two cyclic modes
of progress can be distinguished (Figure 1). At a given point in
time, there is a major unifying configuration, or concept, in a
science which is generally accepted; such a concept will be designated as prejudice. Prejudice generates prediction and experimental action: two consequences follow. Most often, the new experimental results support and develop further the existing prejudice (Mode A progress). On rare occasions, the experimental results obtained are completely unexpected and are of such a fundamental nature that they reveal a paradox (Mode B progress). Paradox, once recognized and generally accepted, leads to tensions and
uncertainty. A variety of new unifying configurations are formu-

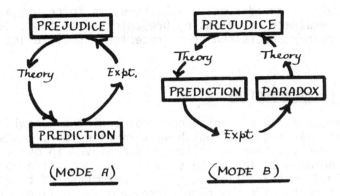

*Figure 1. The relationship between prejudice, prediction, and
paradox in science. Scientific progress occurs via
two cyclic modes, which may be differentiated as Mode
A or Mode B, respectively.*

lated to accommodate paradox. One of these becomes established
as the new prejudice. New predictions are generated and the
cycles repeat. Here I want to make the point that fundamental
theoretical advances occur primarily through Mode B. Each Mode B
cycle penetrates more deeply, approaching, but never achieving, a
final answer. The cycle operates instead to raise new and ever
more fundamental questions. This has been the history of physics
and chemistry; it applies to biology and to the receptor problem
as well. It may be noted, as an aside, in our period of "tight
money" that with each cycle, the costs required to answer the new
questions posed by progress increase markedly, sometimes exponentially.

In this presentation I will attempt to provide an overview of
our current prejudices of hormone research and the receptor concept. I should like to consider where we have come from, and
guess where we may be going. Other participants on this program
will detail the progress achieved in our understanding of the
molecular nature of one or another type of receptor. I look forward to their presentations and know we shall hear the latest com-
muniques from the field of action. What we will hear, I think,
will reflect progress in rapidly changing fields achieved via
Mode A. The new experimental results will clarify, "flesh out,"
and provide new details to support our current prejudices. In
contrast, I shall examine the question whether we may not have
reached a stage in hormone action where paradox exists but is unrecognized. Data which does not neatly "fit" our current prejudices will be examined to determine whether they may represent

the "hints" of the paradox which will come, to force us (as in
chess) to re-evaluate our existing prejudices and, thus, set the
stage for a deeper understanding of receptor structure and function.

Current and Past Prejudices

Our present state of confidence, concerning the newly isolated specific binding units which we term receptors, rests on a
substructure derived from major advances achieved in our understanding of hormone action. The sequence of successive molecular
events involved in the action of sets of hormones and biogenic
amines upon target cells has been worked out in outline form
(Figure 2).

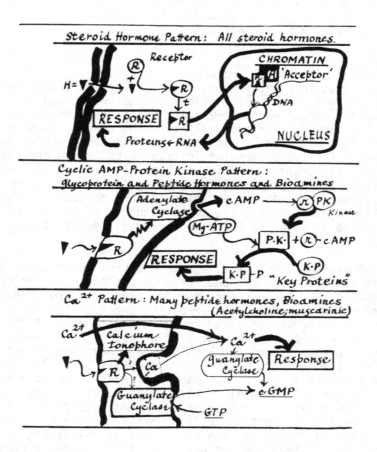

Figure 2.   *Patterns of cellular action; applicable to sets of hormones and/or neurotransmitters.*

Two distinctive patterns of biological action have clearly emerged, which we may now regard as classical. One of these is a pattern applicable to steroid hormones generally; this involves the inter- action of steroid hormone (or active metabolite) with a mobile in- tracellular receptor protein, translocation of the "activated" re- ceptor-steroid complex from the cytoplasm to specific acceptor sites in the chromatin of the nucleus, followed by subsequent mod- ification of genomic activity and protein synthesis. The second classical pattern involves the adenylate cyclase--cyclic AMP-- protein kinase system, applicable to a large number of glycopro- tein and peptide hormones as well as to bioamines, particularly catecholamines. Hormone and neurotransmitter action via the cyclic AMP pattern involves specific receptors localized at the surface membrane of the target cell, "coupled" to adenylate cyc- lase in the same membrane. Recent studies suggest a third pattern involving cyclic GMP and Ca^{2+} (Goldberg, Haddox, Nicol, Glass, Sanford, Kuehl, and Estenson, 1975; Goldberg, O'Dea, and Haddox, 1973). The action of acetylcholine upon "muscarinic" cholinergic receptors is an important example of this pattern. An increasing number of experimental results (*cf.* the review of Berridge, 1975) indicate that the calcium-cyclic GMP pattern most probably involves receptor mediated activation of a membrane unit involved in calcium entry into the cell, the precise nature of which is not known, but which is now popularly considered to be a "calcium ionophore." The increase in cytoplasmic Ca^{2+} produced in this pattern appears to be directly "coupled" to response, Ca^{2+} acting as "second-messen- ger" (*cf.* Rasmussen, Jensen, Lake, Friedmann, and Goodman, 1975); the role of cGMP remains to be elucidated. Many now feel that the increase in cyclic GMP observed in this pattern is a secondary con- sequence of Ca^{2+} activation of cytoplasmic guanylate cyclase (*cf.* Berridge, 1975). It will be recognized that the calcium pattern of biological action is a variation on a very old theme relating to the depolarization of excitable membranes involving Na^+ and K^+. Depolarization (as in the case of acetycholine action upon "nico- tinic" cholinergic receptors) is believed to be achieved via acti- vation of a "Na-K ionophore." Although Na^+ and K^+ are the major ions involved in membrane depolarization, calcium also plays a role in the overall biological response mechanism produced by de- polarization; cytoplasmic Ca^{2+} increases whether due to calcium release from an intracellular reservoir (as in skeletal muscle) and/or as a consequence of increased permeability of the depolar- ized membrane to external calcium.

If we set steroid receptors aside, it will be seen that our current prejudices about receptors, in principle, are not really very different from those enunciated by the pioneers of cell phy- siology and pharmacology, who created the receptor concept at the beginning of this century. We have retained their view that the receptor molecule is the first molecular element of the target cell which "recognizes" a specific extracellular signal (via a selective binding interaction), and then "initiates" a chain of intracellular reactions which leads to response. The receptors of the cyclic AMP pattern and of the calcium pattern correspond to the hypothetical receptors which the creators of the receptor concept had localized at the surface of target cells. The pioneers believed that hormones acted at the surface membrane to control the cellular uptake of ions or substrates (such as glucose) which they considered might be rate limiting for cell function. The ions they felt most likely to be the candidates for participation in hormone action were Na^+ and K^+, in analogy to the depolarization of excitable membranes which they knew something about. Ca^{2+} was added to the "candidate list" in the 1920's, and Heilbrunn at the University of Pennsylvania, vigorously promulgated the view that Ca^{2+} was the "key" to biological action (cf. Heilbrunn, 1956). It is not without interest that our present recognition of the "second messenger" role of Ca^{2+} in hormone action is due in very large part to Howard Rasmussen, also at the University of Pennsylvania (cf. Rasmussen et al., 1975).

Comparing present and past prejudices about receptors, the major change in principle today is our recognition that hormone receptors need not be localized and act at the surface membrane of the target cell. Only the advances achieved with steroid hormone receptors, unexpected in terms of classical prejudice, represent Mode B progress. Our present, more detailed understanding of hormone and transmitter action at the plasma membrane locus represents Mode A progress.

Energetic and Cybernetic Aspects of Receptor Function

The classical receptor concept was developed early in this century when it was traditional to turn to energetics (in the form of thermodynamics or the kinetics derived therefrom) for a set of first principles to explain a biological process. Much of our present approach to receptors derives from and retains this energetic viewpoint in our use of terms like "hormone binding," "amplification," etc. When cybernetics was developed by Norbert Wiener after World War II, an alternative set of first principles to approach certain problems in biology became available. Once it was recognized that molecular genetics could be represented as a set of information transfer reactions, Schwyzer as well as Hechter with associates in the 1960's turned to cybernetics for a set of first principles to understand hormone action. It is not possible here to review the principles of hormone action, (or the related problem of molecular linguistics) which develop from an examination of hormone action from a cybernetic viewpoint (for a recent treatment of the subjects, cf. Hechter and Calek, 1974). It must suffice to state that from a cybernetic viewpoint, hormone (or transmitter) conveys information, in the form of a topochemical pattern, from a "sending" cell to the receptor of the "receiving" cell. The hormonal message is "received" via a pattern recognition reaction, the topochemical pattern of the hormone being "matched" to the topochemical pattern of the receptor. Once received by receptor, the message is "decoded," "transduced" into a new form, and then sent across a "channel" to successive elements of an informational relay system, eventually to reach and "turn on" (or "off") functional "work" units of the cell. The spatiotemporal pattern of effects thus produced constitutes the cellular response appropriate to the original message received. The diagrams in Figure 2 which illustrate the various patterns of hormone action, describe in outline form the "wiring diagrams" of the molecular elements involved in the informational relay systems of three "action programs," each with specific subroutines. The specific action programs are established by genetic instructions; the specific receptors and specific elements which lead to differential cellular responses are likewise "built-in" features of differentiated cells specialized in function. The fact that certain hormones (*e.g.*, thyroxine, insulin, growth hormone) do not really "fit" neatly into one or the other of known "action programs" may be taken to suggest that additional "action programs" remain to be elucidated. Alternatively, it may well be that our presently recognized "action programs" are subroutines of a single master program for regulation of cell function in all its aspects.

One point which emerges from this cybernetic treatment must be emphasized to clarify the receptor concept. The receptor molecule is at once a signal receiver, a signal transducer, and a signal generator (Figure 3). Indeed, the essence of the problem of the receptor transduction function is to define the precise "signal" generated by the receptor-hormone complex (be it chemical or physical in nature), which is sent through a "channel" to the next element(s) in the chain and, likewise, must be defined. This may well be the point to clear up a terminological confusion about the "coupling" process in hormone action. In considering hormone-sensitive adenylate cyclase systems, Rodbell (1971) introduced the idea that a special element designated as transducer, is involved in the process coupling the occupied receptor and the catalytic unit of adenylate cyclase. The "transducer" element has been widely accepted and discussed (*cf*. Perkins, 1973). Rodbell's formulation was developed from an earlier inadequate formulation of this problem where I had introduced the terms "discriminator" for receptor and "signal generator" for the catalytic unit of hormone-sensitive adenylate cyclase systems (Hechter, Yoshinaga, Halkerston, Cohn, and Dodd, 1966). I now recognize that my earlier formulation (as well as Rodbell's amended version) is not consistent with a precise description of receptor function (as shown in Figure 3) whether considered from an informational or energetic point-of-view.

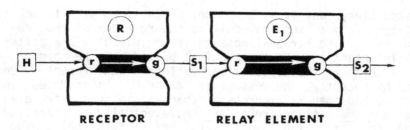

RECEPTOR   RELAY ELEMENT

*Figure 3.   The receptor unit considered from a cybernetic point-
of-view. As illustrated, the receptor (R) molecule is
at once a signal receiver, a signal transducer, and a
signal generator. The occupied receptor upon "activation" generates a new "signal" (S_1) which is sent into
a "channel" and serves to couple the secondary relay
element or effector (E_1) to the "activated" hormone-receptor complex. The "signals" S_1 and S_2 may be either
physical or chemical in nature. The "receiver site"
(r) and the "generating site" (g) of the R and E elements, each of which serves as a transducer, is illustrated. The hormone receptor complex in itself may be
S_1, if it interacts with E_1; alternatively upon occupation, the receptor may either release or produce S_1.*

Current Status of Receptor Isolation

The classical receptor is a bifunctional molecule, which re-
ceives information and then transmits it in another form to a
"secondary" unit. Considered from an energetic point-of-view,
the selective reception of information by a receptor corresponds
to specific binding of hormone by receptor. The availability of
highly radioactive hormones as ligands made it possible to attempt
to identify and isolate receptors by measuring their specific
binding function. It is generally recognized that while all receptors must be specific binding units, all specific binding units
need not necessarily be receptors. Accordingly, certain operational rules have been established to ascertain whether or not the
specific binding units are indeed receptors. These rules, summarized in Table 1, involve six criteria. In general, if the specific binding measured satisfies the first five criteria, the
binding unit is considered to be a receptor in certain journals,
including prestigious journals of biochemistry. Criterion #6 has
rarely been met in reported studies on hormone "receptors." If
Rule #6 were rigidly applied, many of the "hormone receptors" in
the literature would be reduced in status.

Table 1.   *OPERATIONAL RULES USED TO STUDY AND IDENTIFY RECEPTORS*

The general approach has been to measure the "specific" binding
of radioactive hormone (or analog) with appropriate fractions derived from target cells.

Binding ASSUMED to reflect Receptor Interaction, when binding can
be demonstrated to exhibit:

   1.   STRUCTURAL and STERIC SPECIFICITY: Similar to that ob-
        served with a set of analogs.

   2.   SATURABILITY: Limited, finite number of sites.

   3.   CELL SPECIFICITY: in accord with target tissue specifi-
        city.

   4.   HIGH AFFINITY: consistent with physiologic hormone con-
        centration.

   5.   REVERSIBILITY: kinetics consistent with the reversal of
        physiologic effects observed when hormone removed from
        system.

   6.   PARALLELISM between HORMONE BINDING and EARLY CHEMICAL
        EVENT associated with hormone action.

        NOTE: (6) has been demonstrated only in few cases:
                exception not the rule for "receptors" in
                literature.

In this meeting, we will hear studies concerning the isolation and characterization of specific binding units for acetylcholine and certain steroid hormones, which meet the six criteria
set forth in Table 1. Where do we stand with respect to the chemical characterization of these and other receptors? Based upon a
literature survey (which may be incomplete) my best estimate of
the present status of receptor isolation is shown in Table 2; the
degree of purification estimated to be required to obtain pure receptor is shown, together with the degree of purification already
achieved.

Heading the list of reported receptors, is the acetylcholine
receptor (ACh-R) solubilized by detergents from electroplax membranes. Dr. Brady will discuss this receptor in detail. Let me
just state that only about 100- to 500-fold purification is required to isolate the pure receptor from this source (Cuatrecasas,
1974); in 1973, ACh-R had already been isolated in near-homogeneous
form. ACh-R is a macromolecular assembly (about 250,000 to 300,000
M.W.) built primarily of two nonidentical subunits (about 50,000
and 40,000 M.W.). Next is the progesterone receptor from chick
oviduct cytosol; about 4000-fold purification is required to obtain

Table 2. PRESENT STATUS OF RECEPTOR ISOLATION

Receptor (R) and source	Effector to which R is coupled	Purification required for "Pure R"	Purification achieved and results obtained
Acetylcholine (ACh) (electroplax membranes)	Na-K ionophore	100- to 500-fold	Homogeneous R reported: MW about 250,000-300,000 two nonidentical subunits (about 40,000-50,000 MW)
Progesterone (chick oviduct cytosol)	Transcription mechanism (chromatin)	4000-fold	Homogeneous R reported: MW about 23,000 two nonidentical subunits (100,000 and 117,000 MW)
17β-Estradiol (calf uterus cytosol)	"	10^5-fold	Homogeneous "Ca-stabilized form" obtained: (about 78,000 MW)
Gonadotropin (rat testis membranes)	Adenylate cyclase	15,000-fold	Homogeneous R reported: MW about 200,000; subunits ?
[Arg8] vasopressin, glucagon and other small peptides (target cell membranes)	"	about 10^6-fold	Detergent solubilized R obtained: "Near Impossible" to obtain pure receptors at present
Insulin (liver membranes)	several?	about 5×10^5- to 10^6-fold	"

this receptor, according to the report by the group of O'Malley (Kuhn, Schrader, Smith, and O'Malley, 1975). This progesterone receptor is a dimer (225,000 MW) built of two nonidentical sub-units (designated as A and B components), each of which binds pro-gesterone; the role of these subunits in gene transcription will be discussed by Dr. Schrader. To obtain the estradiol receptor from uterine cytosol about 10^5-fold purification is required (Cuatrecasas, 1974) in contrast to 4×10^3-fold purification re-quired for progesterone receptors from chick oviduct. The gonad-otropin receptors in testis membranes which are coupled to adeny-late cyclase have been solubilized by detergents and isolated in pure form (Dufau, Ryan, Bankal, and Catt, 1975); about 15,000-fold purification is required. These receptors are about 200,000 MW; the number and nature of the subunits present has not been deter-mined as yet. Finally to be considered are a set of peptide hor-mone receptors coupled to adenylate cyclase in membranes of vari-ous target cells, as well as the insulin receptor, whose coupling mode in the membrane is not at all clear. Cuatrecasas (1974) has estimated that in order to obtain these receptors in pure form using membranes from conventional target tissue as starting mate-rial, about 10^6-fold purification would be required. It is not surprising that the peptide hormone receptors, some of which have been solubilized from membranes, have not been purified to homo-geneity.

Given this situation, one does not need to be a prophet to predict that the first receptor which will be chemically charac-terized in terms of subunit sequence, will probably be ACh-R from electroplax membranes. Purified ACh-R is already available in milligram amounts; the electric organs necessary as source mate-rial are also available; finally, a large number of effective re-search groups are hard at work on ACh-R. The progesterone re-ceptor from chick oviduct will probably be the second receptor to be characterized chemically. The source material and technics are available; however, funds will be required to set up a "fac-tory" for processing chick oviducts on a pilot plant scale. The gonadotropin receptors from testis would come later; the diffi-culty here is obtaining sufficient source material for pilot plant operation. The possibility of obtaining sufficient pure material for the chemical characterization of peptide hormone receptors seems "near impossible" at this time. New source materials and/or revolutionary new analytical technics must be developed if these receptors are to be isolated and chemically characterized.

If we turn now and consider the state of our knowledge of the effectors to which these receptors must be coupled--a necessary requirement for evaluation of the receptor transducing function-- the situation changes. Indeed, there almost appears to be an in-verse order between the ease of receptor isolation and knowledge of the secondary effector system to which it is coupled. Thus, we perhaps know most about "coupling" in the peptide hormone sensitive adenylate cyclase membrane systems, where we have the greatest difficulty in obtaining pure receptor. This is an embarrassing position since, as previously stated, <u>every</u> specific <u>binding unit need not necessarily be a receptor</u>. Workers in the hormone receptor field should remember the very long controversy as to whether or not acetycholinesterase (whose binding characteristics are very similar to ACh-R) was, in fact, the receptor. Let us, therefore, look critically at some of the specific problems involved in evaluating the <u>transducing function</u> of isolated receptors.

The "Coupling Problem" with ACh-R

ACh-R in electroplax membranes is coupled to a Na^+-K^+ conductance mechanism. This conductance mechanism, once designated as a "channel" or "pore" for Na^+ and K^+, increasingly is now designated as a "Na-K ionophore." E.D.P. DeRobertis (*cf.* DeRobertis, Saez, and DeRobertis, 1975) has proposed a very specific molecular model of the cholinergic receptor, where the "ionophore" is equivalent to a specific channel which develops as the subunits of the receptor separate. Despite extensive knowledge about peptide antibiotics and synthetic molecules which function as ionophores in membranes, there is no general agreement concerning the chemical nature of the specific ionophores <u>intrinsic</u> to excitable membranes or to biological membranes more generally.

The ionophore is <u>the</u> unknown in the ACh-R problem. We know the general principles underlying the action of ionophores which mediate the passage of cations between two aqueous phases separated by a membrane barrier, essentially impermeable to the free cationic species. Ionophores act by interacting with cations to form complexes, soluble in the lipid phase of membranes, which can then traverse the membrane barrier. A variety of intricate maneuvers are intrinsic to this translocation. Ionophores must have the capability for interacting with cations at the interface between one aqueous phase and the membrane; appropriate conformational rearrangements of ionophore are required to permit not only <u>entry</u> of the cation into the interior space, but <u>exit</u> of the cation from the interior space. The known ionophores in chemical terms are small "cage-like" molecules with an "oily" external surface which permits their solubility in nonpolar media, and an internal polar surface into which charged species such as cations can be encapsulated as the ionophore "opens" and "closes." Within the polar interior of the ionophore there must be functional groups (hydroxyl, keto, etc.) with which cations can coordinate. By virtue of such coordinations, it becomes energetically feasible for charged species to shed their water of hydration and form coordinate bonds with the appropriate groups within the interior of the ionophore (Eiseman, Szabo, McLaughlin, and Ciani, 1972).

Dr. Brady will review results suggesting that ACh-R is a polymer built of two primary subunits. Only one of these has binding sites for acetylcholine; the other subunit is widely assumed to represent the elements of the "ionophore." Attractive as this idea may be, there is no compelling evidence that an arrangement of these subunits is, in fact, the ionophore. Highly purified ACh-R electroplax has been available to several groups since 1973. Many attempts have been made to incorporate highly purified electroplax ACh-R preparations into phospholipid bilayer membranes, with the hope of demonstrating increased Na^+ conductance upon addition of acetylcholine (and other appropriate cholinergic agents). The "expected positive finding" has been reported with purified ACh-R preparations from electroplax membranes (Michaelson and Raftery, 1974). Such findings have also been reported with "cholinergic proteolipid" preparations, which DeRobertis and colleagues believe represents ACh-R (for a review of this work, *cf.* DeRobertis *et al.*, 1975), a view not generally accepted by other workers in the field (*cf.* Barrantes, Changeux, Lunt, and Sobel, 1975).

Let us for a moment assume that the "hoped-for" finding in lipid bilayers had been achieved with pure ACh-R. What would this prove? We know that several proteins, completely unrelated to ACh-R may be introduced into "black" membranes and respond to addition of an appropriate ligand by a marked increase in ion conductance. Ligand interaction with a protein in the bilayer which induces a conformational change in the membrane protein modifies the neighboring lipid bilayer arrangement so that ion conductance is increased. One protein which shows this kind of behavior in lipid bilayers is acetylcholinesterase (Jain, Mehl, and Cordes, 1973). Given an experimental setting, where a ligand-induced conformational change of a protein in a bilayer increases ionic conductance, it is not clear to me how study of the incorporation of ACh-R into "black" lipid membranes will precisely define the nature of the "ionophore" intrinsic to the excitable membranes, or the mode of its coupling to receptor. An alternative procedure of elucidating this issue depends upon reconstitution of a chemically excitable membrane (Hazelbauer and Changeux, 1974). Reconstitution of membranes under conditions where purified subunits of ACh-R are used (alone and together) to reassemble ACh-R may resolve the issue. However, there are formidable technical problems raised in such reconstitution experiments. It may well be that defining this coupling problem in ACh-R action will depend upon determining whether a "channel" created by the reaarangement of subunits, or a mobile ionophore is inolved in the conductance event, and by elucidating the chemical nature of ionophores intrinsic to biological membranes.

The "Coupling" Problem in Steroid Hormone Action

It is not possible here to trace the historical developments

which have led to our current picture of steroid action (for a recent comprehensive review of the mechanisms of action of steroid
hormones, *cf*. Liao, 1975). It will suffice to state that the
simplest and currently accepted view of steroid hormone action is
shown in Figure 2. Current prejudice has it that the steroid-receptor complex acts at a nuclear locus to enhance the synthesis of
mRNA that codes for specific protein(s). The mRNA is then required
for the subsequent increase in production of rRNA, and perhaps for
other mRNA species; the latter are translated into proteins, which
then determine the final response. Although the precise mechanisms
of transcriptional control by steroid hormones are a subject of
debate (*cf*. Liao, 1975) there is general agreement that the final
biological response achieved is the consequence of a linear sequence [(steroid-receptor)→DNA→RNA→proteins→"everything else"]
which follows the primary action of the steroid-receptor complex
upon a transcription mechanism.

It has long been apparent that a clear understanding of the
molecular mechanism(s) involved in steroid hormone action must be
dependent on demonstration of the hormonal effect in a simplified
cell-free system. A wide variety of attempts to demonstrate a
clear-cut reproducible effect of receptor-steroid complex on RNA
synthesis in isolated nuclei or chromatin using relatively crude
steroid-receptor preparations have either failed or, at best,
given equivocal results. The purification of the progesterone receptor to homogeneity by the O'Malley group provided material for
a critical test of the idea that the receptor-steroid complex directly acts to influence transcription. Dr. Schrader will present
data that progesterone-receptor complex does, in fact, act *in
vitro* to stimulate the formation of new RNA chain initiation sites
in chick oviduct chromatin. A novel model of steroid hormone action will be presented where one subunit of the steroid-receptor
"dimer" serves to provide the specificity for attachment of the
receptor-steroid complex to specific "acceptor sites" (nonhistone
protein), permitting the second subunit to bind to neighboring
sites on DNA, thus promoting initiation of transcription of specific species of new RNA.

This report from the Houston group, if confirmed, is a major
achievement, whether or not the specific mechanism proposed is
correct in all its details. For purposes of discussion, let us
accept this specific model, not only as established but applicable
to all steroid hormones, so that we may ask the question: "Do we
now understand the molecular basis of steroid hormone action?" I
think the answer must be "No!" It will continue to be no until we
understand how a specific subunit of receptor with steroid "envel-
oped" within a hydrophobic pocket (*cf*. Liao, 1975), once bound to
DNA then acts to "trigger" initiation of RNA synthesis. Is the
protein of the subunit the "actor" in this transduction or does it
merely serve to promote binding to DNA? Does the steroid within

the subunit contribute directly to action, or does it merely serve
an ancillary role serving to hold the protein in the "right" specific conformation? Although there are no answers at present,
these questions must be answered if we are really to understand
the molecular basis of steroid hormone action at the gene locus.

Nor is this our only problem. Steroid hormones can influence
genomic activity and protein synthesis in very different ways (*cf*.
Hechter and Calek, 1974). In differentiation and development,
steroids "switch" the gene program so that one gene set is "turned
on" while another set is "turned off" (*e.g.*, ecdysone in insect
metamorphosis). In other circumstances, steroids may modify a
gene program by introducing one or more genes (via derepression)
into an existing program of "expressed" genes (as with aldosterone
action in the kidney). Finally, steroids may act to influence the
activity of a gene program without necessarily changing gene expression (as appears to be the case with estrogen and androgen
action to maintain the secondary sex organs of mature animals).
What kind of molecular mechanism would provide us with an explanation for so many different consequences of steroid hormone action
at the genomic locus? We will not know until we are able to precisely define the nature of the control mechanisms, operative in
the regulation of gene expression as well as gene activity in eukaryotes.

The difficult issue of gene regulation in eukaryotes is not
the only problem in our understanding of steroid hormone action.
A new complication has developed which raises serious questions
concerning our prejudice that steroids act via the linear sequence
shown in Figure 2. Liang and Liao (1975) have recently shown that
androgens have a dramatic and rapid effect in prostate in regulat-
ing the level of a cytoplasmic protein factor required for initiation of protein synthesis at the ribosomal locus. This ribosomal
initiating factor (RIF) is assayed by measuring the binding of
[^{35}S] methionyl t RNA to the 40 S subunit of the ribosome. One
hour after castration the cytoplasmic level of RIF is decreased;
the depressed RIF level in castrated rats can be increased within
10 minutes after intravenous administration of microgram amounts
of 5 α-dihydrotestosterone (DHT). The DHT effect on RIF is not
blocked by actinomycin D or cyclohexamide; it is blocked, however,
by cyproterone which inhibits the binding of DHT to the androgen
receptor in prostate. Considered together these findings strongly
suggest, but do not prove, that the androgen-receptor complex, independent of its effects at the nuclear transcriptional locus,
acts at another locus in the cell to increase the activity of a
cytoplasmic specific factor required for initiation of peptide
bond synthesis. Indeed, the rapidity of the androgen effect on
RIF, relative to effects on RNA synthesis following androgen administration suggests that the steroid-receptor complex may first
act on the RIF system before nuclear effects on RNA are detected.

In further studies Liao and colleagues (unpublished) have found
that this novel steroid effect is not restricted to the androgen-
prostate system; similar findings with RIF have been obtained in
the estradiol-uterus system as well as the glucocorticoid-liver
system. Thus, the Liao "complication" appears to be a general
feature of steroid hormone action.

Liao's data suggest that the steroid receptor complex acts
at two sites in the cell to coordinate spatially separated functional units involved in protein synthesis, so that the ribosomal
system is "ready" once mRNA species appear in the cytoplasm. With
this finding Liao has opened Pandora's box. Instead of the linear
sequence of Figure 2, the possibility must be considered that the
steroid-receptor complex not only can be shuttled from cytoplasm
to nucleus back to cytoplasm (Liao, 1975), but may act at multiple
loci including the plasma membrane and mitochondria in a coordinated way, so that all requirements for macromolecular synthesis
(including amino acids, glucose, and ATP as well as ions) are
"available at the right time" via a branched reaction sequence shown
schematically in Figure 4. There has always been data in the
steroid hormone field which did not neatly "fit" into the linear
sequence of Figure 2. Some of this data relates to the old idea
that steroids act at the surface membrane of the target cell to
modify transport of glucose and cations (cf. Roberts and Szego,
1953). Recent data supports this idea. Thus, 17β-estradiol (but
not 17α-estradiol) added in vitro to endometrial cells isolated
from rat uterus acts within 1.5 hours to produce significant
changes in glucose metabolism, as well as water and electrolyte
changes, suggestive of sex steroid action at the cell surface
(Pietras and Szego, 1975). Aldosterone, a steroid that is ineffective upon endometrial cells, produced significant effects on
glucose metabolism in epithelial cells isolated from rat urinary
bladder. Pietras and Szego also refer to as yet unpublished
studies which show that estrogen induces alterations in Ca^{2+} binding and/or calcium flux in endometrial cell suspensions. The suggestion that 17β-estradiol may influence Ca^{2+} transport in endometrial cells takes on special significance in relation to reports
that estrogens in rat uterus increase cyclic GMP levels (Kuehl,
Ham, Zanetti, Sanford, Nicol, and Goldberg, 1974) and promote the
synthesis of specific prostaglandins (Ham, Cirillo, Zanetti, and
Kuehl, 1975).

These findings implicating the cell surface serve to remind
us that, about a decade ago, it was reported that high concentrations of gonadal steroids and diethylstilbestrol increased the
flux of ions as well as glucose in liposome membrane systems,
while glucocorticoids reduced these fluxes (Bangham, Standish, and
Weissmann, 1965; Weissmann, 1965). Because of the high concentrations of steroid required, these effects on artificial phospholipid
membrane systems were regarded as of limited physiological signifi-

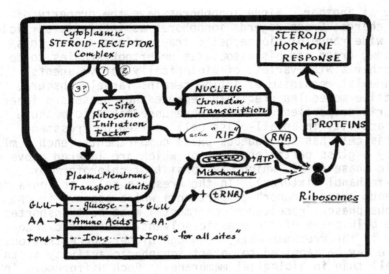

Figure 4.   *Branched sequence of steroid hormone action. An alter-*
native to the presently accepted linear sequence of
steroid hormone action shown in Figure 2. The schematic
illustrates the possibility that the steroid hormone-
receptor complex may act in a coordinated spatiotemporal
pattern at multiple sites in the cell, so that all re-
quirements for macromolecular synthesis are available
"at the right time." In the schematic shown, the
steroid-receptor complex is shown acting first (1) at
an X site to make the ribosomal initiation factor (RIF)
available and then at the chromatin locus (2); the pos-
sibility that the steroid-receptor complex may act at
the plasma membrane locus to activate a set of trans-
port units is shown as (3).

cance. When the field of steroid hormone action developed and
shifted to the genetic locus the issue raised by Weissmann (1965)
was largely ignored. I think that recent studies of David Green
and his associate Godfrey Maina (as yet unpublished) demonstrating
that steroid hormones have ionophoric properties may serve to re-
surrect this issue. Let me tell you how it is that Green came to
examine steroid hormones, and what Maina and Green have found.

For many years David Green has searched for an invariant
principle which underlies energy coupling in all biological systems. His most recent theory (Blondin and Green, 1975) is based
upon the principle that energy coupling requires that paired
charges must be <u>separated</u> at one point in the system and then must

be <u>reunited</u> at another. Since ionophores have the property of separating charge, Green regards ionophores as intrinsic participants in a wide range of bioenergetic transactions. From this point-of-view, Green and his associates undertook studies to determine whether a wide variety of biologically active agents, whose fundamental mechanism of action remains largely obscure, might be active molecules precisely because they possessed inherent ionophoric properties. Studies were undertaken to measure ionophoric activity in an all-glass cell devised by Pressman (1973). This cell has two aqueous phase compartments (each 2 ml) separated by a glass partition, both of which are layered above a bulk organic phase (6 ml, which may consist of chloroform or chloroform-methanol mixtures). In the Pressman cell, an ion added to one aqueous phase ("donor" compartment) which appears in the other aqueous phase ("receiver compartment") must be transported through the bulk phase of the organic solvent. Authentic ionophores work in the Pressman cell, although higher concentrations of ionophore may be required to detect ionophoric activity in the Pressman cell than in biological membranes. Such differences in the effective ionophore concentrations required are not surprising, when it is considered that ionophore is shuttling ions across a 75° A lipid barrier in a membrane and across several centimeters of bulk organic solvent in a Pressman cell.

The foregoing serves as an introduction to the preliminary results obtained by Maina and Green. They tested a limited number of steroid hormones and analogs for ionophoric activity in the Pressman cell adding ^{45}Ca to the "donor compartment" and measuring radioactivity in the "receiver compartment" [which contained EDTA (125 mM) and citrate (50 mM)]. Steroid hormones were added to the organic phase [chloroform-methanol (2:1)]. None of the natural steroid hormones exhibited ionophoric activity for ^{45}Ca when the donor compartment contained $CaCl_2$ at neutral pH. However, when 5 mM inorganic phosphate (Pi) was added to the "donor" compartment containing $CaCl_2$, all of the steroid hormones now exhibited clear ionophoric activity as measured by appearance of ^{45}Ca in the receiver compartment, <u>presumably because ^{45}Ca and P_i were transported together by a steroid ionophore system.</u> Under the specific conditions used, the transport units varied from about 30 to 2 nanomoles of ^{45}Ca per micromole steroid per hour transported from "donor" to "receiver" compartment.

The most active ionophores under the conditions tested were testosterone and progesterone (about 30 units); the least active was aldosterone (about 2). The relative effectiveness of steroid hormones as ionophores appeared to be inversely related to the polarity of the steroid molecule and had the order: testosterone= progesterone>corticosterone>17β estradiol>aldosterone. In contrast to steroid hormones, cholesterol was found to be essentially inactive as an ionophore. For myself, the striking and unexpected finding in the Green-Maina study is that steroid hormone specificity was exhibited in the Pressman cell. 17β-estradiol was found to be about 100-fold more effective than its inactive stereoisomer (17α-estradiol); in contrast, diethylstilbestrol and ethinylestradiol were found to be equivalent to 17β-estradiol in ionophoric activity. Cyproterone, the androgen antagonist, is not only active as an ionophore, but may perhaps be more effective than testosterone or 5α-dihydrotestosterone.

The preliminary findings of Maina and Green, which I have presented, are just the beginning of a project where much remains to be done. A wide variety of steroid analogs of the androgen, estrogen, progestin, and corticosteroid series must be systematically examined with divalent metals (M^{2+}), including Mg^{2+}, Mn^{2+}, and Ca^{2+} as well as monovalent cations. The role of anions, other than P_i (capable of "working with" metals at neutral pH) in the Pressman cell, must also be studied. Only then will it be possible to assess the relationship between ionophoric activities of these steroids. I do not know what results will emerge, nor do I know the physiological significance of such results once obtained. However, these striking results of Maina and Green have "forced" me to think about the possible significance of steroid "ionophores." Let me "think out loud" and share my speculative fantasies with you.

In order for a steroid hormone to function as an ionophore in the Pressman cell, where the bulk organic phase consists of a chloroform-methanol mixture (saturated with water), it is necessary to postulate that steroid molecules must assemble (via intermolecular hydrogen bonding) to form a "cage-like" structure with a nonpolar exterior and a polar interior, in order to fulfill the fundamental structural features required for ionophoric activity. The individual steroid molecule with rigid conformation cannot meet these structural features. Within the polar interior of the "cage-like steroid polymer" the "free" polar groups of the steroid hormone assembly must be appropriately arranged spatially so that the ions involved (Ca^{2+} and P_i) can be coordinated to multiple polar sites; the differences in ionophoric activity observed between 17β- and 17α-estradiol are explicable only on this latter basis. Turning from the Pressman cell to a target cell responsive to steroid hormones, what can one say about steroid ionophoric activity in the living cell? The obvious possibility is that steroids may assemble in biological membranes (whether alone or with phospholipids and/or protein elements) to form the ionophores intrinsic to biological membranes capable of transporting "ion pairs" (e.g., Ca^{2+} and P_i) into the cell. Less obvious, but more interesting, are the new possibilities which arise when one considers steroids "ionophores" in relation to steroid-receptor proteins. Consider, the situation which arises when a single steroid hormone molecule is "enclosed" within the "hydrophobic pocket" of a

protein subunit of the receptor (*cf.* Liao, 1975). In this case we
may assume that the polar groups at one end of the steroid molecule together with CO, NH, and OH elements (from backbone as well
as amino acid sidechains) at the surface of the receptor pocket
may be <u>spatially arranged within the hydrophobic pocket</u>, so that
coordination of metal (M^{2+} with or without an anion) becomes possible on a 1:1 molar basis. Such a receptor-steroid-metal complex,
if it were "fixed" in the plasma membrane, might account for ster-
oid-induced transport changes. However, there is a second possibility which I find intriguing. A receptor-steroid-metal ternary
complex which is mobile in the cytoplasm would have the capacity
to shuttle M^{2+} selectively to M^{2+} <u>binding sites</u> throughout the
cell, provided that these M^{2+} binding sites are associated with
"acceptor sites" which interact with the protein of the receptor-
steroid complex. If the "acceptor" protein has M^{2+} binding sites
its interaction with steroid-receptor-M^{2+} complex might result in
transfer of M^{2+} from <u>receptor</u> to "<u>acceptor</u>." If the M^{2+} binding
sites are associated with a critical molecule neighboring the "acceptor," interaction of receptor with "acceptor" might release M^{2+}
so that it is available for a "critical" M^{2+} binding site. In
either case, the steroid-receptor complex might serve to shuttle
M^{2+} to specific M^{2+} binding sites on specific molecular species
which are critically involved in the functional response, not only
in the chromatin of the nucleus but throughout the cell. On this
view, for example, steroid hormone action at a plasma membrane
locus would be due to the interaction of steroid-receptor-metal
complex with plasma membrane "acceptor sites" of units associated
with the transport of glucose, cations, amino acids, etc. Such a
mechanism might well provide the basis for the coordinated response pattern, shown in Figure 4, which is operative over a period of hours, during which time receptor in its various complex
forms may recycle between cytoplasm and nucleus.

It will be recognized that the postulated steroid-receptor-
metal complex is <u>not</u> an ionophore in the classical sense of the
term, <u>which implies shuttling ions within a membrane</u>; here it
serves as a mechanistic device for shuttling metals (without or
with anions, *e.g.*, phosphate) to specific critical sites throughout the cell involved in the spatiotemporal sequence of biological
action. The nature of the specific metals transported by the postulated receptor-steroid-metal complex, over a period of hours, may
involve Mn^{2+}, Mg^{2+}, and Ca^{2+}. It is not unattractive to consider
that the Mn^{2+} and Mg^{2+} required for RNA polymerase activities
might be "taken" to nuclear sites by a steroid-receptor-metal complex at the same time that the receptor complex "triggers" initiation of transcription. It is possible, for example, to consider
that the interaction of receptor steroid-Mg^{2+} complex with the
critical binding sites on an "acceptor" may involve an exchange reaction (say Ca^{2+} for Mg^{2+}), so that a newly formed receptor-steroid-

Ca^{2+} complex no longer can bind to nuclear "acceptor sites," and thus returns to the cytoplasm. And one could go on!

It is apparent that a wide variety of new possibilities arise from the concept that receptor-steroid complexes may serve as devices for the shuttle of ions to specific critical sites in the cell. The elements of the idea, it will be recognized, are merely a variation on a basic theme employed in the calcium pattern of biological action. The major difference is the manner in which the M^{2+} "signal" is conveyed to the functional response units. In the conventional calcium pattern, the response mechanism is sensitive to the level of cytoplasmic Ca^{2+}; "excitation" (whether produced by hormones of bioamines) produces a rapid "pulse" of free Ca^{2+} which is recognized by sensitive regulatory proteins (e.g., troponin) which act to "turn on" the system; other elements which lower cytoplasmic Ca^{2+}, whether by sequestering calcium in reservoir systems (sarcoplasmic reticulum, mitochondria, etc.) or by promoting Ca efflux act then to turn the response mechanism "off." In contrast, steroid hormone action involves a spatiotemporal series of coordinated reactions extending over hours, not seconds or minutes: coordinated control involving the cell "as a whole," can not be achieved by simply increasing M^{2+} for protracted intervals over many minutes or hours. Moreover, the special requirement for steroid hormone action to influence a small number of specific genes in the genome poses a requirement for localized effects (involving nearest neighbors in a small micro-environment) which cannot be achieved by raising (or lowering) the concentration of M^{2+} throughout the nucleoplasm.

I should warn you that the speculation advanced concerning the receptor-steroid-metal shuttle is a modern version of an old idea presented many years ago at the First International Congress on Hormonal Steroids (Hechter, Halkerston, and Eichhorn, 1964). There I presented a paper on cortisol action and suggested that divalent cations (Ca^{2+} in particular) might be released from the steroid receptor, at one stage or another, to "trigger" the sequence of molecular arrangements we recognize as response. I do not know whether the present proposal that receptor-steroid complex serves as a device for shuttling metals to critical sites is any better in 1975 than it was in 1964. The major difference is that technology is available today to subject this idea to experimental analysis. Whether the concept advanced today is correct or untenable, in whole or in part, will only be established by future experiments. I should tell you, however, that the primary purpose of this speculative exercise is to illustrate the extreme fragility of our current prejudices in steroid hormone action and to show how rapidly, once paradox appears, one can conceive new and more inclusive concepts about steroid hormone action.

The Coupling Problem in Hormone Sensitive Adenylate Cyclase Systems

The problem here is to define how a receptor in the plasma membrane, upon interaction with a specific protein hormone or transmitter, activates a protein enzyme (adenylate cyclase) in the same membrane. A wide variety of specific models have been proposed to account for "coupling" in hormone sensitive cyclase systems (cf. the mini-review of Boeynaems and Dumont, 1975). It is not possible here to review these proposals, except to note that there is no compelling evidence which forces acceptance of one coupling model to the exclusion of others.

One problem is that the molecular nature of receptor and adenylate cyclase is not known in detail; the spatial relationship, as well as the stoichiometry of receptor and enzyme units in the membrane, is likewise unknown. The molecular arrangement of these elements is a central issue in the elucidation of the coupling process because completely different types of mechanisms are required, depending upon whether or not receptors are structurally contiguous to enzyme units. If the units are coupled structurally as well as functionally, certain mechanisms are likely; if the receptor and cyclase units are spatially separated within the membrane, other mechanisms must be invoked to "connect" these elements functionally. In the past, it was assumed by many that the discrete units of adenylate cyclase systems are coupled structurally (via noncovalent bonding). With the recognition that membrane proteins are free to diffuse laterally within the "lipid sea" of a Singer-Nicolson (1972) type membrane, a new possibility for coupling receptors and enzymes has become popular. In one view it takes the form that receptor and enzyme of adenylate cyclase systems are initially spatially separated, but that following interaction of hormone with receptor the HR complex migrates through a "fluid" membrane to interact with enzyme (E) to form a ternary complex [H-R-E], which is regarded as the activated form of the enzyme. This "two-step" fluidity hypothesis for coupling has been promulgated with great vigor by Cuatrecasas (1974, 1975).

To illustrate the nature of specific technical problems encountered when one tries to define the nature of the coupling process in hormone sensitive adenylate cyclase systems, I propose to discuss in some detail the neurohypophyseal hormone (NHH) sensitive cyclase systems in renal medullary membranes which have been extensively studied for years. The NHH-responsive system in pig membranes has been particularly well characterized in an important series of publications by the group of Jard, Bockaert, Roy, and associates at the College de France (for a review, cf. Jard, Roy, Barth, Rajerison, and Bockaert, 1974). This group has provided substantial evidence that the specific ^{3}H-LVP binding sites in porcine renal medullary membranes, first detected by Campbell, Woodward, and Borberg (1972), have the specificity and kinetic charact-

eristics expected for functional NHH receptor coupled to adenylate
cyclase. The receptor sites detected by binding studies behaved
as a homogeneous population of molecules with a single affinity
constant for ^{3}H-LVP. After detailed study of the properties and
characteristics of the receptor and adenylate cyclase units in
porcine membranes, they studied the coupling process by measuring
the relationship between ^{3}H-LVP binding and enzyme activation under identical experimental conditions, where steady-state enzyme
stimulation had been achieved and binding was at or near equilibrium. Under these "steady-state" conditions, a nonlinear relationship was observed between receptor occupancy and enzyme activation. Submaximal concentrations of ^{3}H-LVP which occupied only
10% of the receptor sites produced a disproportionate degree of
enzyme activation (40%-80% of maximal enzyme stimulation depending
upon the Mg^{2+} concentration in the medium). Maximal enzyme activation, however, was achieved, only with hormone concentrations
which occupied all of the receptor sites. The observed nonlinear
relationship between hormone occupancy and enzyme activation implied that occupation of a small fraction of receptor sites by low
hormone concentrations activated multiple catalytic units; with
stepwise increase of hormone concentration the "multiplication
factor" in coupling progressively decreased, so that at maximal
hormone concentrations there is a 1:1 relationship between occupation and activation.

What is the nature of this nonlinear coupling process operative in the NHH-sensitive adenylate system? Let me try to answer
this question on the basis of our own studies on the NHH-sensitive
adenylate cyclase system in bovine renal medullary membranes. I
will take you rapidly through several years of work, to provide
the background material for the studies on bovine membranes to be
described. We used a partially purified plasma membrane preparation derived from the renal medulla of heifers; plasma membranes
were purified using a polyethylene glycol-dextran double phase
method (Nakahara, Pincus, Flouret, and Hechter, manuscript in
preparation). Tritiated lysine vasopressin (^{3}H-LVP), arginine
vasopressin (^{3}H-AVP), and oxytocin (^{3}H-OT) were synthesized (via
tritiation of the diodo derivatives) and subsequently purified (by
neurophysin-sepharose columns and other chromatography procedures)
to radiochemical homogeneity; the tritiated hormone preparations
had specific activities which ranged from 20 to 30 Ci per mmole
(Terada, Nakagawa, Hechter, and Flouret, in preparation). Specific
binding of H-LVP and receptor-mediated cyclase activation in bovine membranes were measured under identical experimental conditions so that for each hormone concentration studied, activation
(A) could be related to occupation (O). The standard incubation
conditions employed for assay of specific binding and NHH-adenylate
cyclase activity (corrected for basal activity) involved membrane
incubation under conditions which <u>minimize</u> basal adenylate cyclase

activity and <u>maximize</u> the ratio of NHH-sensitive cyclase activity
to basal activity. Basal activity in renal medullary preparations
is due to the basal activities of a multiplicity of adenylate
cyclases derived from the heterogeneous cell types in renal medulla, most of which do not respond to NHH: the conditions selected
thus permit study of the NHH-specific cyclase system with minimal
"background noise." Membranes are incubated at 30°C in a medium
with 25 mM Bis-Tris propane (pH 8.5), 2.0 mM $MgCl_2$, 1.4 mM EDTA,
100 µM ATP, 1 mM cyclic AMP, 20 mM creatine phosphate, and 0.2 mg
per ml creatine kinase. The bovine membranes were shown to be de-

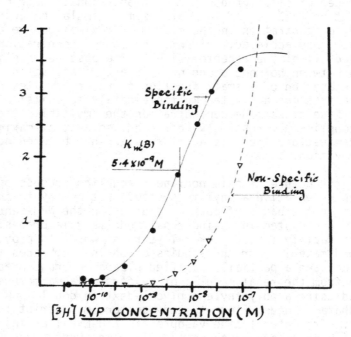

*Figure 5.   Specific and nonspecific binding of ³H-LVP in bovine
renal medullary membrane preparations. Results obtained
with a typical bovine membrane preparation incubated at
30°C for 15 minutes with various concentrations of [³H]-
LVP (both in the presence and absence of 10⁻⁵ M unlabeled LVP) at which time [³H]-LVP binding is at or near
equilibrium. Binding was measured with a Millipore
technic. Specific binding is the difference between
total binding (absence of 10⁻⁵ M unlabeled hormone) and
the ³H-LVP binding which occurs in the presence of 10⁻⁵
M unlabeled LVP (nonspecific binding). The units of
binding are expressed in p/moles ³H-LVP bound per mg
membrane protein.*

void of enzymatic activity capable of degrading ^{3}H-LVP or ^{3}H-OT; the radioactivity recovered from membranes after incubation with ^{3}H-LVP or ^{3}H-OT for 60 minutes consisted of a single peak on several thin-layer chromatography systems with mobility identical to the standard tritiated hormone.

Bovine renal medullary membranes have specific binding sites for ^{3}H-LVP (Figure 5). In six different preparations, the total number of specific binding sites varied from 1.3 to 3.9 pmoles ^{3}H-LVP per mg membrane protein. The ^{3}H-LVP concentration required for half-maximal binding [$K_m(B)$] likewise varied from one preparation to another, ranging from 4 to 19 nM. Scatchard analysis of ^{3}H-LVP binding in all preparations showed a linear plot; the Hill coefficient was near 1.0 (ranging from 0.94 to 1.06). These observations indicate that the specific sites in bovine membranes detected by ^{3}H-LVP binding, like those in porcine membranes, appear to be homogeneous with respect to affinity and that binding is noncooperative. The specificity of the binding sites by ^{3}H-LVP in bovine membranes was determined by competitive binding studies with a set of unlabeled NHH analogs, which differ profoundly in antidiuretic activity and have different apparent affinities for activation of bovine NHH adenylate cyclase. These studies (Hechter, Terada, Spitzberg, Nakahara, and Flouret, in preparation) showed that the specific binding sites have the specificity characteristics expected for functional bovine renal NHH receptors coupled to adenylate cyclase. Figure 6 shows the striking linear relationship between the peptide concentration required for half-maximal adenylate cyclase activation and for specific binding (as estimated from competitive binding studies; *cf.* Figure 7).

Having reasonable evidence that the specific ^{3}H-LVP binding sites correspond to functional NHH-receptor units, the coupling process was studied by measurement of hormone occupancy of sites and adenylate cyclase stimulation under "near equilibrium" conditions. The effects of various concentrations of ^{3}H-LVP on adenylate cyclase activity was measured over a 5-minute interval, 12.5 minutes after hormone addition, when enzyme stimulation had reached "steady-state." ^{3}H-LVP binding was measured at 15 minutes, at which time binding is at or near equilibrium. The coupling process in bovine membranes under these conditions may be defined in terms of the A:O relationship "normalized" so that total ^{3}H-LVP binding and maximal NHH adenylate cyclase activity are both set at 100%. Figure 8 shows the nonlinear A:O relationship obtained in bovine membranes which is similar to that previously described in the porcine membrane system, (Jard *et al.*, 1975). This nonlinear A:O normalized relationship was strikingly similar in different bovine membrane preparations, despite three-fold differences in the total number of specific binding sites and the fact that the ratio of receptor sites/maximal enzyme activity ranged from 1.6 to 5.8 (arbitrary units). Despite differences suggesting variable ratios

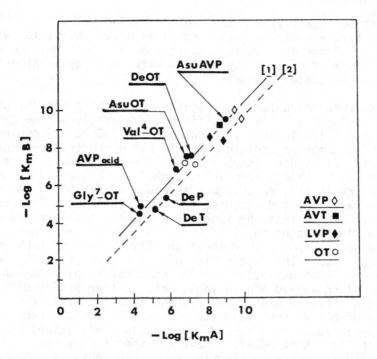

Figure 6. *Comparison of the apparent affinities of natural neuro-hypophyseal hormones and a set of synthetic analogs for binding and for activation of adenylate cyclase. The peptide concentration required for half maximal specific binding $[K_m(B)]$ and half-maximal activation of NHH-specific adenylate cyclase $[K_m(A)]$ was determined in two bovine membrane preparations, under standard conditions. The $[K_m(B)]$ and $[K_m(A)]$ values for unlabeled peptides were obtained under "steady-state" conditions. The abbreviations used are: Arg^8 vasopressin (AVP), $[Lys^8]$ vasopressin (LVP), $[Arg^8]$ vasotocin (AVT), Oxytocin (OT), deaminoxytocin (DeOT), deminopressinamide (DeP), deaminotocinamide (DeT), Aminosuberic (Asu). The $[K_m(B)]$ value for LVP was directly determined using ^3H-LVP; the $[K_m(B)]$ values for the other peptides were calculated from H_{50} values for the unlabeled peptides in competitive binding studies with ^3H-LVP (as shown in Figure 7). The linear relationship between the parameters for this set of peptide agonists indicates that the specific membrane sites detected with ^3H-LVP binding are the same sites as those involved in adenylate cyclase activation. In six different membranes the ratio of $[K_m(B)]/[K_m(A)]$ for ^3H-LVP ranged from 3.1 to 6.2. The $[K_m(A)]$ values were likewise consistently less than the $[K_m(B)]$ values with AVP and OT as well as NHH analogs.*

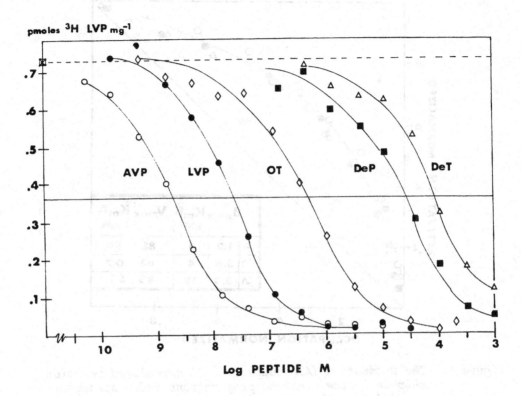

Figure 7. The specificity of the specific membrane sites detected by [³H]-LVP binding, as determined by competitive binding studies. In the experiment shown above, the [³H]-LVP concentration (1.26 x 10⁻⁸M) employed, occupied 60% of the total binding sites in the absence of unlabeled peptides. The effect of addition of various concentrations of unlabeled peptides upon [³H]-LVP binding was determined 15 minutes after simultaneous addition of unlabeled peptide and [³H]-LVP. Knowing the $K_m(B)$ value for [³H]-LVP and the concentration of unlabeled LVP necessary to reduce [³H]-LVP binding by 50% (H_{50}), it is possible to calculate $K_m(B)$ values for each of the peptides studied, from the H_{50} values on the basis that the unlabeled peptide competes with the labeled ligand for all of the specific binding sites. A large variety of unlabeled peptides (including angiotensin II, glucagon, insulin, ACTH[1-24], and ACTH[1-10]) tested at concentrations as high as 3 x 10⁻⁴ did not influence [³H]-LVP binding.

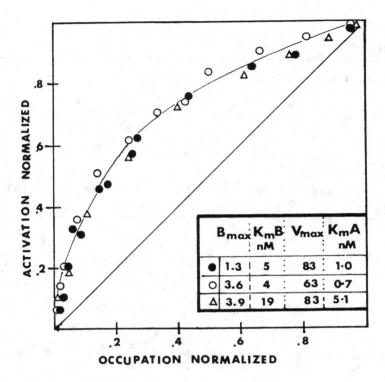

*Figure 8.   The activation (A)-occupation (O) normalized relation-
ship in bovine membrane preparations under steady-state
conditions.   The A:O normalized relationship is similar
in different bovine renal medullary membranes despite
differences in these preparations in the ratio of total
number of specific [³H]-LVP binding sites (Bₘₐₓ in units
of pmoles [³H]-LVP bound/mg protein) to the maximal NHH-
cyclase activity (Vₘₐₓ in units of pmoles cAMP mg/pro-
tein/per minute).*

of receptor units and catalytic units in these bovine membranes,
the "steady-state" A:O normalized relationship in all membranes
showed the feature that at 4% occupancy the A:O ratio was about 5;
at 10% occupancy the A:O ratio decreased to about 4, and then
further as occupation increased.   When ³H-AVP is used in similar
experiments, the A:O normalized relationship is similar to that
observed with ³H-LVP.   Alteration of incubation conditions (whether
by change in pH, by addition of inhibitors such as 2.0 mM $CaCl_2$, or
by 0.1 mM GTP) which produce a marked decrease in maximal NHH
cyclase activity and/or ³H-LVP binding capacity (and/or affinity)

does not essentially modify the shape of the "steady state" A:O normalized relationship. The nonlinear coupling process in bovine membranes thus appears to be "shielded" from the action of external agents which may profoundly modify receptor behavior and/or the catalytic activity of the enzyme. The "stability" of the nonlinear coupling process strongly suggests that coupling may be an intrinsic feature of membrane organization, relating to a specific pattern of molecular arrangement of receptor and catalytic units.

Having observed that the A:O "steady-state" normalized relationship was remarkably similar in membranes with different ratios of ^{3}H-LVP binding sites/maximal NHH-cyclase activity, the detailed dynamics of ^{3}H-LVP binding and enzyme stimulation was studied in two membrane preparations with identical maximal NHH-cyclase activities (82 pmole cAMP/min/mg) which differed 3-fold in the total number of specific ^{3}H-LVP binding sites (1.3 and 3.9 pmole ^{3}H-LVP bound/mg); [$K_m(B)$] for ^{3}H-LVP was 5 mM and 19 mM for the "low R" and "high R" membranes, respectively. The dynamic results obtained were very different for these two membrane preparations, but were internally consistent for each preparation (Figure 9). In the "high R" membrane, hormone binding and activation of adenylate cyclase followed a similar time course with the four submaximal ^{3}H-LVP concentrations studied (and with five ^{3}H-AVP concentrations not shown); both of these parameters reached "steady-state" at about the same time. Thus, in this membrane, hormone occupation of receptor sites appeared to be directly related to enzyme activation as previously reported for the porcine membrane system (Brockaert, Roy, Rajerison, and Jard, 1973). The time course for binding and enzyme stimulation observed in the "low R" membrane differed from that in the "high R" membrane. The discrepancy between hormone occupancy and enzyme activation was progressively greater as ^{3}H-LVP concentration was increased. With high ^{3}H-LVP concentrations in the "low R" membrane, steady-state enzyme activation occurred before binding equilibrium; ^{3}H-LVP binding continued after steady-state enzyme velocity had been achieved until equilibrium binding was obtained. The receptors in the "low R" membrane behaved as if they were "programmed" to recognize and respond to a given initial hormone concentration by rapidly "recruiting" and "activating" a fixed multiple number of catalytic units, in such a way that other receptor units become "silent."

Given excellent kinetic data on two membrane systems, both well characterized in terms of specific binding sites and NHH adenylate cyclase activity, how does one explain the differences observed in the dynamic A:O normalized relationship? The unexpected finding in the "low R" membrane suggesting a programmed receptor response to a given initial concentration of hormone, raised the possibility that a specific geometric relationship between receptor (R) and catalytic (C) units could be formalized such that a probabilistic model could be developed to account for the variable

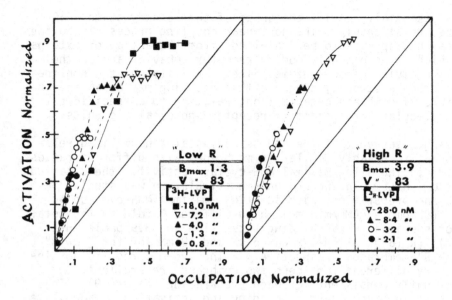

Figure 9.   *The dynamic A:O normalized relationship in two membrane*
preparations with identical V_{max}, which differ 3 fold
in B_{max}.   Two well characterized bovine membrane prepa-
rations designated as "high R" and "low R" with identi-
cal V_{max} (83 pmoles cAMP mg^{-1} $min.^{-1}$) but differing in
B_{max} (3.9 and 1.3 pmole ^3H-LVP bound mg^{-1}) were incu-
bated with varying concentrations of ^3H-LVP.   The ki-
netics of ^3H-LVP binding and adenylate cyclase activa-
tion were studied under identical dynamic conditions
starting 30 seconds after hormone addition.   It will be
seen that the dynamic A:O normal relationship obtained
is strikingly different in the "low R" and "high R"
membrane preparations.

multiplication factor in coupling as well as the increase in "silent receptors" observed as hormone concentration is increased.
The problem is to arrange R and C units in such a way that the
model <u>predicts</u> the dynamic and steady-state normalized A:O response
of the "lower R" membrane.   This problem was discussed with a number of theoretical biologists.   What follows is a probabilistic
model developed by Dr. Richard Bergman (Department of Biomedical
Engineering, University of South California), an experimental endo-
crinologist who happens to be a gifted theoretician.

We assume that R and C units are present in equal number and
arranged in "fixed" 20 x 20 matrices within certain regions of the

membrane as shown in Figure 10. Ignoring edges, each unit of the
R matrix is in "contact with" five C units in the lower matrix;
the C unit immediately below the given R unit and the four nearest
neighbors of that C. The C units are identical and are considered
to be in one of two idfferent states: "active" or "inactive." The
R units are identical and are considered to be in one of two different states: "occupied" or "unoccupied." We assume that in a
matrix where all R units are unoccupied, the first "effective"
collision of a hormone molecule with a R unit generates a signal $\underline{S}$
which, after a certain time interval, activates five nearest neighbor C units (cf. Figure 10). Depending upon hormone concentration,
which determines the rate at which hormone-receptor interactions
occur, it is apparent that as the R matrix is progressively "filled,"
the probability increases that hormone will interact with R units
where some and then all of the associated nearest-neighbor C units
are already in activated state. Hormone occupation of such a R
unit would have no effect on enzyme stimulation so that such hormone binding would appear to be "silent."

Bergman simulated the behavior of this model on a digital computer. He has been able to predict the dynamics of hormone occupation and enzyme activation which occur in this model as the number
of effective collisions per unit time (a parameter which is directly related to hormone concentration) is systematically varied, as-
suming an exponentially distributed occupancy time for R units
and a distribution of delay times between occupation and activation of C units. The simulated dynamic curves for hormone binding
and enzyme activation have precisely the form as the actual data
obtained with different ^{3}H-LVP concentrations in the "low R" membrane preparation. The model also successfully predicts the nonlinear relationship observed between hormone concentration and the
A:O normalized ratio, both transient and in steady-state.

Having a model which accounts for the "unexpected" dynamic A:O
response in the "low R" membrane, how does one account for the dissimilar normalized dynamic response in the "high R" membrane? Can
the matrix model successful in one case be applied to the second,
so that we can account for membrane differences in the dynamic A:O
response and still obtain an essentially similar A:O relationship
in the steady-state? As mentioned previously, the two membranes
have identical NHH specific cyclase activity but differ 3 fold in
the number of receptor sites. The model shown in Figure 10 assumes
a 1:1 relationship of R and C units. If such a relationship applied in the high R membrane, then to account for the identity of
the normalized A:O relationship in steady-state, it would be necessary to assume either that (1) the catalytic capability of the C
units are reduced; (2) the transient coupling characteristics are
different; or (3) both of the above. In effect, since the dynamic
normalized A:O relationships are clearly different, the high R

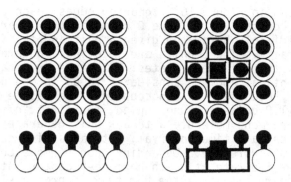

*Figure 10.   Interlocking coupled matrix model for arrangement of
receptor (R) and catalytic (C) units within a region
of the plasma membrane. The schematic illustrates a
section of a 20 x 20 matrix of R units overlaying a
20 x 20 matrix of C units. The R units are identical
and exist in one of two states: unoccupied (●) or occupied (■); the C units are identical and exist in one
of two states: inactive (o) or active (□). Each R
unit is assumed to be coupled to five "nearest-neighbor" C units, so that hormone occupation of a given R
unit after a characteristic delay activates five C
units (provided that they are in an "inactive state").
In the schematic above, a R unit once occupied by a
hormone molecule activates five C units in the "overlap" pattern described in the text. During the interval in which the R unit illustrated is still occupied,
its "nearest-neighbors" R sites could only activate
three C units if they were "hit." This model successfully predicts the normalized A:O relationship observed
in the "low R" membrane preparation both for the dynamic and steady-state response. The matrices for R and C
units are drawn to show "top" and "edge" views "before"
and "after" a single R site is occupied. The left side
of the schematic shows the state before hormone; the
right side is the state after a single hormone molecule
has filled one R site. In the "edge view" of the schematic, the unoccupied R units are shown attached to C
units by a "stalk." Upon hormonal occupation the R
unit "contracts" into a "compressed state," in contact
with 5 C units. The specific structural arrangement
of R and C units shown is not a unique feature of the
model, but serves to illustrate one possible way by
which an occupied R unit is able to activate a multiple
number of "nearest-neighbor" C units. Alternative
possibilities of achieving activation of 5 C units by
occupation of a single R unit are described in the
text.*

membrane must be viewed as differing either in geometric organization of elements (R:C ratio, 3:1) and/or in the characteristics of
the coupling process.

    There are several simple geometric possibilities for the ar-
rangement of R and C units on a 3:1 basis. The high "R" membrane
may have 1225 R units in a 35 x 35 matrix, associated with 400
"effective" C units, the remaining C units being either uncoupled
or denatured in the course of membrane purification. The C units
can be arranged either at random or in clusters, so that a limited number of R units each has the possibility of activating 5 C
units. We may also consider the situation where there are 1200 R:
400 C with the C units arranged in a 20 x 20 matrix. In one arrangement, R units may be packed "on top of" the 20 x 20 matrix
so there are 3 R units per C unit, with each R having an equal op-
portunity of interacting with nearest-neighbor C units of the matrix. Alternatively, the extra R units may be arranged in the
membrane such that the standard 20 x 20 matrix of C units is inter-
locked with a 20 x 20 of R units, and the extra R units (*ca.* 800)
are arranged in a membrane section which is spatially separated
from the coupled matrices of R and C units (Figure 11). Computer
simulation of the normalized A:O relationships which develops in
all of these diverse geometric arrangements fails to predict the
differences in normalized enzyme activation relative to normalized
occupation observed with the "high R" membrane.

    Given the fact that no simple geometric construction can ac-
count for the dynamic differences between the "high R" and "low R"
membranes, we were left with the possibility that there is a significantly longer delay time for coupling in the "high R" membrane
than in the "low R" case. By increasing the time required for
coupling in the "high R" membrane, it became possible on computer
simulation to account for the differences in the dynamics of the
normalized A:O relationship between membranes while retaining the
similarity of the steady-state normalized A:O relation. It is to
be emphasized that the effect of modifying the coupling delay upon
the transient normalized A:O behavior is independent of assumptions
concerning the stoichiometric relationship of R and C units.

    In effect, with three assumptions: (1) that R and C units are
arranged on a 1:1 basis in an interlocking matrix arrangement, (2)
hormone occupation of R results, after characteristic time periods,
in activation of a variable number of C units, the maximal number
being 5 C units, and (3) the delay in coupling may vary between
membranes, it is possible to account for the paradoxical differences
observed in the coupling behavior of these two different membrane
preparations in terms of straightforward probabilistic collision

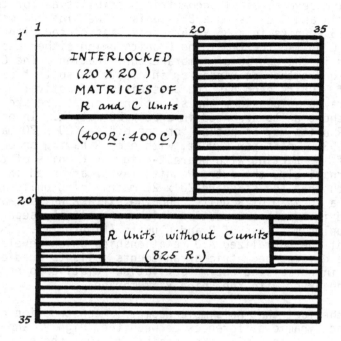

Figure 11.   An arrangement of R and C units in a membrane where
             the stoichiometric relationship of R to C units is
             3:1.   In the schematic shown above, 400 C units are
             arranged with 1225 R units in two discrete regions of
             the membrane.   In one region, 400 R units are arranged
             in a 20 x 20 matrix interlocked with a 20 x 20 matrix
             of C units (as in Figure 10), with occupation-activa-
             tion characteristics previously described.   The remain-
             ing 1024 R units are arranged in another region of the
             membrane devoid of C units, thus occupation of these
             latter units has no influence on adenylate cyclase ac-
             tivation.   This model, as well as all other geometric
             arrangements of R and C units on a 3:1 basis, fails to
             predict the dynamic normalized A:O relationship ob-
             served in the "high R" membrane.

theory. This theoretical analysis of hormone receptor interaction
in relation to coupled enzyme activation is now being prepared for
publication (Bergman and Hechter, in preparation).

The specific model proposed has a wide variety of implications
relating to the molecular organization of receptors and coupled
enzyme units within membranes as well as to the questions of "silent" receptors, "multi-valent" adenylate cyclase systems (where
multiple receptors appear to be coupled to the same catalytic
unit), etc., but this is not the place to discuss these issues.
Instead, I should like to consider which features of the matrix
model presented should be regarded as fundamental. The size and
shape of the matrices of the model are not fundamental; any interlocking coupled matrix system involving a sufficient number of R
and C units which provides for the fundamental overlap feature of
the model would be adequate. Similarly, the specific packing arrangement which provides for maximal activation of 5 C units per
initial R unit occupied is not fundamental; alternative packing
arrangements of R and C units within matrices are possible so that
six (or more) units of C are activated by occupation of one R (via
hexagonal or other packing arrangements of units). A fundamental
feature of the present model is that there be a delay in coupling
so that activation of a multiple number of nearest-neighbor C units
does not occur instantaneously upon occupation. Coupling must involve a time-dependent process, where the C units are activated
in sequence rather than in concerted fashion. The model as drawn
shows a type of structural coupling between R and C units of two
matrices relatively fixed in space, but this feature is not unique.
The R units need not be arranged in a "rigid" matrix structurally
contiguous to the C units of a rigid matrix. The R units may be
mobile above a relatively fixed matrix of C units, and vice versa,
but a restricted "interaction field" for R units must be maintained.
The model postulates only two states for R and C units; transition
states are ignored. Nevertheless, we know there are at least three
states for R units: unoccupied, occupied-inactive (as with competitive inhibitors), and occupied-active. With adenylate cyclase,
there are likewise multiple transition states (Rodbell, Lin,
Salomon, Londos, Harwood, Martin, Rendell, and Berman, 1975). Accordingly, while the present data and the matrix model presented
do not exclude other possibilities, the present model accounts for
"coupling" in terms of a probabilistic theory of hormone interaction
with receptors with a minimal number of *ad hoc* assumptions.

The question which is left open by our model, and this is the
central issue in the coupling problem, is how an R unit once occupied, after a characteristic delay, activates a multiple number of
neighboring C units. There is substantial evidence that a guanine
nucleotide, which acts at a nucleotide regulatory site on the enzyme, may perhaps be involved as an intermediate in the activation

of adenylate cyclase (Rodbell *et al.*, 1975). Whether a nucleotide itself is the coupling signal S or modifies the rate of appearance of S remains to be elucidated. In either case, a problem remains: how can the interaction of certain topochemical
elements of a peptide hormone molecule with complementary elements
within a hydrophobic pocket at the exterior of a receptor unit (of
MW about 100,000-200,000) produce effects at a distance (say 20°-
30°A) upon nearest-neighbor enzyme units, whether directly or in-
directly via a nucleotide? Based upon our recent studies of
retro-D-analogs of oxytocin (Hechter, Kato, Nakagawa, Yang, and
Flouret, 1975) we had suggested that a unique topochemical arrangement of the CO elements of the peptide backbone might be
critically involved in the "activation" of receptors by oxytocin
and, perhaps, for peptide hormones more generally. Having previously raised the issue that a steroid hormone enclosed within
the "pocket" of a receptor may serve to provide for an arrangement of multiple polar groups for coordination of metal (say Ca^{2+}
and/or Mg^{2+}), I cannot now help wondering whether the "trigger" of
the peptide hormone receptor complex may not likewise involve a
metal. On this view, the elements of the peptide backbone of the
hormone would play a critical role in the coordinate bonding of a
metal within a hydrophobic pocket of the receptor. A conformational change in a receptor unit which brings a coulombic charge provided by M^{2+} into a nonpolar matrix of catalytic units might well
serve as the "trigger" which is "propagated" and "spreads" to the
nearest neighbors to initiate action, with or without nucleotide
participation.

What I have just suggested is a variation of an old theme in
peptide hormone action discussed by peptide chemists for many
years. I first heard this view from Josef Rudinger, how deceased,
who thought that peptide hormone action might involve a metal-pep-
tide complex required for both binding and activation of receptors;
for oxytocin and a number of other peptides, the "key" metal might
be Mg^{2+} and/or Mn^{2+}; for ACTH, MSH (and the related peptides of
this family) the "key" metal might be Ca^{2+}; for angiotensin, perhaps Na^{2+}. I must confess, that while at that time I "heard"
Rudinger, I did not really "listen."

Summary

Major progress has been achieved in understanding the chemical
nature of receptors for certain hormones and neurotransmitters.
Some of these units have been obtained as homogeneous proteins;
concept and technology are adequate to permit the detailed chemical
and structural analysis of these macromolecular units. The critical problem which now arises is to define how a receptor once "occupied" and "activated" serves to initiate action. Elucidation of
details of receptor structure, in of itself, will not solve the

"coupling problem" in hormone action. New concepts, as well as new technics, will probably be necessary. In this discussion I have raised the possibility that metals coordinated to hormone receptor complexes may be the "trigger" element involved in initiating action, serving to alter the state of functional units in binary fashion. In effect, the metal determines whether the "state" of the system is <u>active</u> or <u>inactive</u>. As stated previously in connection with the action of steroid hormone receptor complexes, the specific suggestions made relating metals to the hormone coupling process have been advanced primarily to illustrate the conceptual gap which exists with respect to "coupling." The present suggestions may prove to be correct or untenable, in whole or in part. If it turns out that metals play a central role in the coupling process of hormone action, perhaps via completely different mechanisms than those suggested here, one of the central ideas of receptor action developed by the pioneers who created the receptor concept will have been resurrected in principle, if not in detail. In science, as in life generally, conceptual progress once achieved sometimes turns out to be the rediscovery of the past.

REFERENCES

Aurbach, G.D. (1975) Beta-adrenergic receptors, cyclic AMP and ion transport in the avian erythrocyte. *J. Cyclic Nucleotide Res.* 5:117-132.

Bangham, A.D., Standish, M.M., and Weissmann, G. (1965) The action of steroids and streptolysin S on the permeability of phospholipid structures to cations. *J. Mol. Biol.* 13:253-259.

Barrantes, F.J., Changeux, J.P., Lunt, G.G., and Sobel, A. (1975) Differences between detergent-extracted acetylcholine receptor and "cholinergic proteolipid." *Nature* 256:325-327.

Berridge, M.J. (1975) The interaction of cyclic nucleotides and calcium in control of cellular activity. *Adv. Cyclic Nucleotide Res.* 6:1-98.

Blondin, G.A. and Green, D.E. (1975) A unifying model of bioenergetics. *Chem. and Eng. News* 53(45):26-42.

Bockaert, J., Roy, C., Rajerison, R., and Jard, S. (1973) Specific binding of [^{3}H] lysine-vasopressin to pig kidney plasma membranes: Relationship of receptor occupancy to adenylate cyclase activation. *J. Biol. Chem.* 248:5922-5931.

Boeynaems, J.M. and Dumont, J.E. (1975) Quantitative analysis of the binding of ligands to their receptors. *J. Cyclic Nucleotide Res.* 1:123-142.

Campbell, B.J., Woodward, G., and Borberg, V. (1972) Calcium-mediated interactions between the antidiuretic hormone and renal plasma membranes. *J. Biol. Chem.* 247:6167-6175.

Cuatrecasas, P. (1974) Membrane receptors. *Ann. Rev. Biochem.* 43:169-214.

Cautrecasas, P. (1975) Hormone receptors--their functions in cell
    membranes and some problems related to methodology. *Adv.*
    Cyclic Nucleotide Res. 5:79-104.
Cuatrecasas, P., Jacobs, S., and Bennett, V. (1975) Activation of
    adenylate cyclase by phosphoramidate and phosphonate analogs
    of GTP: Possible role of covalent enzyme-substrate intermed-
    iates in the mechanism of hormonal activation. *Proc. Nat'l.*
    Acad. Sci. USA 72:1739-1743.
DeRobertis, E.D.P., Saez, F.A., and DeRobertis, E.M.F., Jr. (1975)
    Molecular biology of receptors. In: *Cell biology* (6th ed.),
    pp. 564-568, W.B. Saunders Co., Philadelphia.
Dufau, M.L., Ryan, D.W., Bankel, A.J., and Catt, K.V. (1975)
    Gonadotropin receptors: Solubilization and purification by
    affinity chromatography. *J. Biol. Chem.* 250:4822-4824.
Eisenman, G., Szabo, G., McLaughlin, S.G.A., and Ciani, S.M. (1972)
    Molecular basis for the action of macrocyclic carriers on
    passive ionic translocation across lipid bilayer membranes.
    Bioenergetics 4:295-350.
Goldberg, N.D., O'Dea, R.F., and Haddox, M.K. (1973) Cyclic GMP.
    Adv. Cyclic Nucleotide Res. 3:155-223.
Goldberg, N.D., Haddox, M.K., Nicol, S.E., Glass, D.B., Sanford,
    C.H., Kuehl, F.A., Jr., and Estensen, R. (1975) Biologic
    regulation through opposing influences of cyclic GMP and
    cyclic AMP: The Ying Yang hypothesis. *Adv. Cyclic Nucleo-*
    tide Res. 5:307-351.
Ham, E.A., Cirillo, V.J., Zanetti, M.E., and Kuehl, F.A., Jr.
    (1975) Estrogen-directed synthesis of specific prostaglandins
    in uterus. *Proc. Nat'l. Acad. Sci. USA* 72:1420-1424.
Hazelbauer, G.L. and Changeux, J.P. (1974) Reconstitution of a
    chemically excitable membrane. *Proc. Nat'l. Acad. Sci. USA*
    71:1479-1483.
Hechter, O. and Calek, A. Jr. (1974) Principles of hormone action:
    The problem of molecular linguistics. *Acta Endocrinol.* 191:
    39-66.
Hechter, O., Halkerston, I.D.K., and Eichhorn, J. (1964) The mode
    of action of cortisol upon lymphocytes. In: *Hormonal*
    steroids, biochemistry, pharmacology and therapeutics. Pro-
    ceedings of the First International Congress on Hormonal
    Steroids 1:359-374.
Hechter, O., Kato, T., Nakagawa, S.H., Yang, F., and Flouret, G.
    (1975) Contribution of peptide backbone to the action of
    oxytocin analogs. *Proc. Nat'l. Acad. Sci. USA* 72:563-566.
Hechter, O., Yoshinga, K., Halkerston, I.D.K., Cohn, C. and Dodd,
    P. (1966) Hormone action in relation to the generalized
    problem of intercellular communication. In: *Molecular basis*
    of some aspects of mental activity (O. Wallas, ed.) Vol. 1:
    291-346, Academic Press, New York.
Heilbrunn, L.V. (1956) *Dynamics of living protoplasm.* Academic
    Press, New York.

Jain, M.K., Mehl, L.E.,and Cordes, E.H. (1973) Incorporation of
    eel electroplax acetylcholinesterase into black lipid mem-
    branes: A possible model for the cholinergic receptor.
    Biochem. Biophys. Res. Comm. 51:192-197.
Jard, S., Roy, C., Barth, T., Rajerison, R., and Bockaert, J.
    (1975) Antidiuretic hormone-sensitive kidney cyclase. *Adv.*
    Cyclic Nucleotide Res. 5:31-52.
Kuehl, F.A. Jr., Ham, E.A., Zanetti, M.E., Sanford, C.H., Nicol,
    S.E., and Goldberg, N.D. (1974) Estrogen-related increases
    in uterine guanosine 3':5'-cyclic monophosphate levels.
    Proc. Nat'l. Acad. Sci. USA 71:1866-1870.
Kuhn, R.W., Schrader, W.T., Smith, R.G., and O'Malley, B.W. (1975)
    Progesterone binding components of chick oviduct X: Purifica-
    tion by affinity chromatography. *J. Biol. Chem.* 250:4220-
    4228.
Liang, T. and Liao, S. (1975) A very rapid effect of androgen on
    initiation of protein synthesis in prostate. *Proc. Nat'l.*
    Acad. Sci. USA 72:706-709.
Liao, S. (1975) Cellular receptors and mechanisms of action of
    steroid hormones. *Internat'l. Rev. Cytol.* 71:87-172.
Michaelson, D.M. and Raftery, M.A. (1974) Purified acetylcholine
    receptor: Its reconstitution to a chemically excitable mem-
    brane. *Proc. Nat'l. Acad. Sci. USA* 71:4768-4772.
Perkins, J.P. (1973) Adenyl cyclase. *Adv. Cyclic Nucleotide Res.*
    3:1-64.
Pietras, R.J. and Szego, D.M. (1975) Steroid hormone-responsive
    endometrial cells. *Endocrinology* 96:946-954.
Pressman, B.C. (1973) Properties of ionophores with broad range
    cation selectivity. *Fed. Proc.* 32:1698-1703.
Rasmussen, H., Jensen, P. Lake, W., Friedmann, N., and Goodman,
    D.B.P. (1975) Cyclic nucleotides and cellular calcium metab-
    olism. *Adv. Cyclic Nucleotide Res.* 5:375-394.
Rodbell, M. (1971) Hormones, receptors and adenyl cyclase activ-
    ity. In: *Colloquium on the role of adenyl cyclase and*
    cyclic 3':5' AMP in biological systems (P. Condliffe and M.
    Rodbell, eds.), pp. 88-95, Fogarty International Center,
    Government Printing Office, Washington, DC.
Rodbell, M., Lin, M.C., Salomon, Y., Londos, C., Harwood, J.P.,
    Martin, B.R., Rendell, M., and Berman, M. (1975) Role of
    adenine and guanine nucleotides in the activity and response
    of adenylate cyclase systems to hormones: Evidence for
    multisite transition states. *Adv. Cyclic Nucleotide Res.* 5:
    3-30.
Roberts, S. and Szego, C.M. (1973) Steroid interaction in the
    metabolism of reproductive target organs. *Physiol. Rev.* 33:
    593-629.
Schramm, M. (1975) The catecholamine-response adenylate cyclase
    system and its modification by 5'-guanylimidophosphate. *Adv.*
    Cyclic Nucleotide Res. 5:115.

Singer, S.J. and Nicolson, G.S. (1973) The fluid mosaic model of
     the structure of cell membranes. *Science* 180:968-971.
Weissmann, G. (1965) Lysosomes. *N. Engl. J. Med.* 273:1084-1090.

DISCUSSION AFTER DR. HECHTER'S PAPER

Dr. DeGroot
Are your results from the vasopressin studies compatible with the models of adenylcyclase floating around the membrane and occasionally winding up at the receptor?

Dr. Hechter
The two-step fluidity hypothesis for receptor coupling, advanced independently by Contrecasas and De Haen, postulates that R and C units are free to "float" in the lipid sea of a Singer-Nicolson type membrane. The hormone-receptor complex (HR) when formed is assumed to have high affinity for cyclase (C), and diffuses through the lipid to interact with C to form a ternary (1:1:1) complex, considered to be the activated form of the enzyme. Our matrix model suggests that the R and C units are not structurally coupled (via noncovalent binding), but are clustered in certain regions of the membrane. Although the units are free to "move," they do so only within certain restricted fields. Thus, a single occupied R is free to interact with, and thus activate, a multiple number of "nearest neighbor" C units, provided that they are in an inactive state. A maximum of 5 C units may be activated by a binding event at a single R unit in our model, but free diffusion of the occupied R unit outside its restricted "interaction field" is excluded. There is a further requirement that the interaction of the occupied receptor with C units must occur in a temporal sequence so that the individual coupling delays must be exponentially distributed. Accordingly, while our model has certain features which are similar to the "floating receptor" idea, it differs with respect to the stoichiometry of the interaction of HR with C units, and particularly in the restrictions placed on the lateral diffusion of R and C units in the membrane.

Dr. Campbell
Have you ever reached the limit on nonspecific binding in your membranes? Saturation of nonspecific binding must be difficult to achieve.

Dr. Hechter
In our bovine renal medullary preparations, we have never been able to saturate the nonspecific binding sites either with tritiated lysine vasopressin (LVP), arginine vasopressin (AVP), or oxytocin (OT). Nor do we know whether these sites are present primarily in the membrane fragments from cell types not responsive to ADH or from ADH-responsive cells in the distal nephron and collecting tubules. We have not been able to separate plasma membrane fragments with vasopressin receptors from the plasma membrane fragments without these receptors. Our efforts to apply affinity chromatography to purify NHH-responsive membranes have so far failed. Given

heterogeneity of membrane elements, I am not sure what nonspecific
LVP binding means. It should be mentioned that the set of neuro-
hypophyseal hormones we use are peptides which in high concentration are disulfide reagents, capable of interacting with thiol
groups on a membrane, via a thiol-disulfide interchange reaction.
There are additional interaction possibilities between peptides
and surfaces, which contribute to nonspecific binding, so that it
is difficult to know what nonspecific binding actually measures.

Dr. Freed

I would like to point out that in your Mode A and Mode B of
scientific advancement, in Mode A whenever possible there should
be branchings in the generation of predictions from experiments,
and a Mode B situation actually arises when those branchings that
are important go unrecognized.

Dr. Hechter

Let's get together, so that you can help me change the figure
appropriately.

Dr. Barnawell

I'd like to ask a practical question; then a physiological
question. First, you mentioned the fact that when you used freshly synthesized lysine vasopressin, unless I misunderstood you,
that only lasts for about three months. You mean you have to re-
synthesize new, dry peptides each time?

Dr. Hechter

Are we talking about labelled or unlabelled hormone?

Dr. Barnawell

Unlabelled. I keep it dry in the freezer over desiccant and
make it up in solution fresh when I'm using it. Does this seem
like a safe procedure?

Dr. Hechter

In our experience with neurohypophyseal peptides, we find
that dimerization and polymer formation is minimized when the
powders are dissolved in water containing trace acid (acetic or
formic acid) and stored as aliquots at -70°. "Dry" powders, may
have tightly bonded water, and are not necessarily dry.

Dr. Barnawell

I could use that one. My physiological question is: I can
sympathize with your choice of cells which allow you to see what
you're looking for, but I fail to understand why there are neurotransmitter receptors on red blood cells or even on liver cells.
I don't really understand any biological function for such receptors on these cells.

Dr. Hechter
I have ideas about the issue you raise, but they represent nothing more than my personal philosophical prejudices, and I'm sure that others have alternative prejudices which, likewise, are not compelling. Given this situation, I am not sure that this is the place to discuss the philosophy of biology.

Mr. Morgan
I'm sure you're aware of the recent literature about some enzymes that are found on membranes which seem to degrade the peptide hormones responsible for activation of adenylate cyclase, in particular, lysine vasopressin. Do you have any way of including the kinetics of that reaction?

Dr. Hechter
The bovine renal medullary membranes that we use do not degrade either tritiated AVP, LVP, or OT. We see no evidence of hormone metabolites in the medium by thin-layer chromatography. If you isolate the bound peptides from membranes, there is likewise no evidence of any metabolic transformation. Accordingly, we feel degradative enzymes are not a necessary feature of the action of these peptides in our membrane preparations.

Dr. Campbell
In the Fitzpatrick membrane preparation (Fitzpatrick *et al.*, 1969, *J. Biol. Chem.* 244:3561), there's an ATP-dependent calcium uptake. Do you see any relationship between this and the mechanism of action of the hormone?

Dr. Hechter
We have no information on this point.

Dr. Siegel
Dr. Hechter, as a student of molecular linguistics, in your model you used the term prejudice rather than dogma, is that deliberate?

Dr. Hechter
Dogma has a transcendental theological connotation which I would not apply to prejudice.

Dr. Siegel
I think it's quite clear from this very provocative and very comprehensive presentation that the notion of receptors, while very helpful, is still making it even more elusive as to what the true nature of hormonal action really is. In fact, I fear the analogy of the onion is still very, very applicable to contemporary endocrinology. Every time we peel another layer of onion we still get tears, there's another layer to go, and yet when will we really get to the heart of the onion?

NUCLEAR RECEPTORS FOR THYROID HORMONE

L.J. DeGroot

Thyroid Study Unit, Dept. of Medicine
University of Chicago
Pritzker School of Medicine
Chicago, IL   60637

INTRODUCTION

The concept that thyroxine (T_4) or triiodothyronine (T_3) might act by modification of nuclear RNA synthesis was advanced by Tata in the early 1960's (Tata, Ernster, and Suranyi, 1962). He reported that T_4 induced new RNA and protein synthesis, and indicated later that the earliest observable effect was on the function of nuclear magnesium-dependent polymerase involved in ribosomal RNA synthesis (Tata and Widnell, 1966). An effect was observed 12 hours after administration of hormone to hypothyroid rats. In 1966, Cohen reported that T_4 treatment augmented template function of tadpole liver chromatin (Kim and Cohen, 1966), and Tabachnick reported binding of thyroid hormone to histone from calf thymus nuclei (Tabachnick and Giorgio, 1966).

T_3 Nuclear Receptors -- *in Vivo* Experiments

The first demonstration of "specific" T_3 binding sites in animal tissues occurred in 1972. Oppenheimer and coworkers reported the presence of binding sites for the hormone in pituitary (Schadlow, Surks, Schwartz, and Oppenheimer, 1972), liver, and kidney (Oppenheimer, Koerner, Schwartz, and Surks, 1972). T_3 was found to equilibrate within a period of three hours in the pituitary and reached at equilibrium a concentration in the pituitary of approximately ten times that of blood at the same time interval. In-

*Supported by United States Public Health Service Grants AM-13,377, CA-14,599, and AM-17,310.

45

creasing doses of T_3 caused apparent saturation of the binding
sites. Estimated capacity was in the order of 12 ng/g pituitary,
and it was believed that the binding sites were normally fully
saturated at existing plasma levels of the hormone. T_3 appeared
to bind with about ten times the affinity of T_4 to these sites.
Rat liver and kidney also contained receptors which could be saturated with increasing doses of hormone injected *in vivo*. These
workers suggested that the sites were relatively specific for T_3
and did not bind T_4. Binding sites in the cytosol were recognized
and found to be nonsaturable under the conditions of the experiment.

During 1972, Philip Cohen and coworkers reported the distribution of T_4 injected into tadpoles and found that the material
was accumulated over two hours in the nuclei of animals maintained at 25° C, but little entered the nuclei if animals were maintained at 5° C (Griswold, Fischer, and Cohen, 1972). The T_4 was
found bound tightly to chromatin, and was not chemically altered
during the *in vivo* experiments reported. The hormone was not removed from the nuclei after washing with 0.05% Triton X-100 to
remove the outer nuclear membrane and was, surprisingly, not separated from chromatin when the nuclei were broken in EDTA solutions and then washed with 0.3 M KCl. (This treatment solubilizes
liver nuclear T_4-binding protein, *v.i.*) Cytosol binding proteins
for T_4 were also recognized in the tadpole liver preparations.

Our own studies on T_3-binding sites in rat liver nuclei began
in 1972, but were initially fraught with difficulty. Using the
method of Blobel and Potter (1966) for preparation of liver nuclei
in Tris-potassium chloride-magnesium chloride and sucrose (TKMS),
we were unable to demonstrate the presence of saturable nuclear
binding sites. On switching to the .32 M sucrose + 1 mM magnesium
chloride homogenization solution used by other investigators, it
was easily possible to reproduce their results. At first this
finding appeared strange, but we have since recognized that it was
due to extraction of the nuclear binding proteins from the nuclei
during homogenization and centrifugation in the TKMS buffer system. Nuclear T_4 binding protein is soluble in salt solutions and
its distribution between "cytosol" and nuclei depends upon the
method of tissue preparation utilized.

Rats were given I^{125}-T_3 *in vivo* and then killed two hours
later. Approximately 9% of liver isotope was present in the nuclear fraction prepared by centrifugation of a 1,000 x g crude
nuclear fraction through a sucrose gradient (DeGroot and Strausser,
1974). Equilibration of injected T_3 between serum cytosol and nuclei occurred within one to two hours. Peak ratios of nuclear T_3
to total liver T_3 occurred at 3.5 hours, but remained relatively
constant over 24 hours as T_3 was metabolized and cleared by the
animal. Liver/serum T_3 isotope ratios were approximately 4.5 at

two hours after injection of the isotope. In hypothyroid rats, nearly twice as much of the isotope was present in the nuclei when tracer quantities were injected. When increasing doses of stable T_3 were injected with the labelled T_3, saturation of the binding sites was achieved in both normal and hypothyroid animals at approximately the same level of injected hormone. The T_3 injected in $vivo$ and bound to liver nuclei could be displaced by injecting unlabelled T_3. Triodothyroacetic acid (Triac) was, surprisingly, found to have equivalent (or greater) ability to displace the T_3 from nuclear receptors. L-T_4 was less active and D-T_4 was even less active in displacing T_3. Capacity of the binding sites in nuclei was approximately 2.4 ng T_3/g liver in hypothyroid animals. Since normal rat nuclear T_3 content was about 0.6 ng/g, the binding sites were normally occupied to the extent of about 25% of saturation in $vivo$.

During incubation of nuclei (labelled with T_3 in $vivo$) in $vitro$ at 37° C, it was found that T_3 eluted from the nuclei, especially in the presence of protein-containing solutions. This indicated that T_3 was bound reversibly and that there was dissociation of the T_3 from nuclear T_4 binding protein and/or the T_3-receptor complex from the nuclear chromatin. We also found that the material present in the nuclei could be extracted with 0.4 M KCl and migrated in sucrose gradient with a Svedberg constant of 4S. The extracted nuclear binding protein-T_3 complex was destroyed by pronase, but not by RNAse or DNAse, indicating its protein nature.

Extensive studies on the kinetics of binding were reported by Oppenheimer and coworkers in 1974 (Oppenheimer, Schwartz, Koerner, and Surks, 1974). Equilibrium distribution of T_3 appeared to occur between cytosol, nucleus, and serum within one-half hour. Rat serum T_3 content was 0.84 ng/ml. Nuclear T_3 binding capacity was 1.6 ng T_3/g liver, and they estimated that binding sites were normally approximately 70% saturated. The binding affinity for T_3 was reported to be 13- to 24-fold greater than the affinity for T_4. The association constant of T_3 for the nuclear sites was approximately $5 \times 10^{11} M^{-1}$ (Table 1), as determined in their in $vivo$ experiments.

One study has reported the T_3 binding capacity of various rat tissues (Oppenheimer, Schwartz, and Surks, 1974). The capacities, in comparison to liver, are given in Table 2. Capacity descends in an approximate order of pituitary-liver-kidney-heart-brain, with spleen and testis being the lowest. In this study endogenous liver T_3 was found to be about 1 ng/g tissue and percent saturation of tissue binding sites averaged approximately 50%. The binding affinity of the sites for T_3 was found to be similar in all tissues, although there were marked differences in binding capacity.

Table 1. BINDING OF T_3 TO RAT LIVER RECEPTORS *IN VIVO*

Tissue	Ka	Capacity ng/g liver	Capacity ng/mg DNA	Normal % saturation	Estimated sites/nucleus	Authors
Hypothyroid Rat Liver		2.4			10,400	DeGroot & Strausser, '74
Normal Rat Liver	$4.7 \times 10^{11} M^{-1}$	1.6	.52	70%	4,400	Oppenheimer, Schwartz, Koerner, & Surks, '74

Table 2. NUCLEAR T_3 BINDING CAPACITY OF VARIOUS RAT TISSUES

	Endogenous T_3 ng/mg DNA	Binding capacity ng/mg DNA	tissue/liver	ng/g	tissue/liver	Percent saturated
Liver	.61	.61	1.0	1.77	1.0	47
Brain	.27	.27	.44	.42	.24	39
Heart	.4	.4	.65	.8	.45	44
Spleen	.018	.018	.03	.31	.18	50
Testis	.002	.0023	.004	.022	.01	90
Kidney	.5	.53	.87	2.61	1.47	35
Pituitary	.79	.79	1.3	6.58	3.72	48

(From Oppenheimer *et al.*, 1974.)

The nature of the nuclear T_3 binding material was investigated by DeGroot and coworkers (DeGroot, Refetoff, Strausser, and Barsano, 1974). Rat liver nuclei were labelled by *in vivo* administration of ^{125}I-T_3 and then extracted *in vitro* with 0.4 M KCl, 1 mM magnesium, and 10 mM sodium phosphate buffer, pH 7.4 (KMP). Increasing concentrations of salt (such as KCl), ranging from .05 to .4 M, extracted progressively more of the labelled nuclear T_4 binding protein-T_3 complex from nuclei. Increasing pH also augmented recovery of the material. The binding characteristics of the nuclear T_4 binding protein-T_3 complex were studied by incubation of the complex with Dowex-1 anion exchange resin, which bound free T_3, but not the T_3 complexed to protein. Usually 50% of the T_3 recovered from the nuclei was found complexed to a protein, and 50% behaved as if it was free T_3. The complex was thermolabile and was inactivated at 50°-70° C within a few minutes. It was also destroyed by pronase or urea, and by incubation with 0.1-1 mM parachloromercuribenzoate (PCMB). During electrophoresis the nuclear T_4 binding protein-T_3 complex migrated anodally in a broad band. The T_3 bound to the protein did not exchange readily with unlabelled T_3 at 0° C. This complex, incubated *in vitro* with chromatin, rebound to chromatin at low KCl concentrations, but not at high salt concentrations. Thus, the material was a protein with a negative charge at pH 8, bound to nuclear components in a noncovalent manner, bound T_3 in a thermolabile manner, and had a required sulfhydryl group. Affinity for chromatin was demonstrated by the rebinding experiments.

In a similar study, Surks, Koerner, Dillman, and Oppenheimer (1973) found that the nuclear T_4 binding protein complex present in rat liver nuclei was not removed by Triton X-100 washing of the nuclei, but was extracted with high salt concentrations, and was associated with chromatin. They suggested that T_4 bound primarily to the outer nuclear membrane and this binding was largely nonspecific. The nature of the complex was studied in their laboratory using gel filtration chromatography with Sephadex G-50; results indicated that it was a macromolecule. They noted thermolability at 25-37° C and confirmed the sensitivity of the protein to pronase but not to DNAse or RNAse. The molecular weight of the complex was 60,000-70,000 and the concentration of rat plasma T_3 was reported to be 1.29 pmols/ml and T_4 59 pmols/ml; nuclear T_3 was 0.72 pmols/g, and T_4 was 0.43 pmols/g. These authors reported that iodoacetate, mercaptoethanol, dithiothreitol, and glycerol did not stabilize the nuclear T_4 binding protein-T_3 complex.

T_3 Receptors in Isolated Nuclei

Binding of T_3 and other hormone analogs to nuclei or cells *in vitro* has been investigated in a number of laboratories, and results are fairly consistent. Variations are probably accounted for by differences in tissue preparation and incubation conditions in the individual studies (Table 3).

In our own laboratory, rat liver nuclei were prepared by homogenization and sedimentation of the nuclear fraction through sucrose, and incubation *in vitro* usually in a solution of 0.32 M sucrose, 1 mM magnesium, 10 mM pH 7.85 Tris-HCl buffer (SMT) with 5 mM dithiothreitol (DeGroot and Torresani, 1975). In this system the K_d for T_3 was $5 \times 10^{10} M^{-1}$ and binding capacity was approximately 0.5 ng/g liver. Optimal binding was observed at 20° C, although binding did occur at 0-2° C, and much more rapidly at 37° C. Binding was similar at pH 7.85 and at pH 7.4, and was significantly augmented by including dithiothreitol in the medium. We believe dithiothreitol protected the relatively unstable nuclear T_4 binding protein-T_3 complex from aerobic inactivation. The addition of calcium enhanced nuclear integrity but reduced T_3 accumulation. EDTA and phosphate caused nuclear damage but, perhaps for this reason, augmented T_3 accumulation by nuclei. The process of binding of T_3 to nuclei did not require generation of high energy phosphates and was not inhibited by puromycin or actinomycin D. Binding did not require the mediation of a cytosol protein and, therefore, seemed to occur by free T_3 complexing directly with binding sites in the nucleus. The binding was obliterated by pronase, but not by RNAse or DNAse. The addition of from 5-50 mM sodium or potassium did not alter binding. The nuclear T_4 binding protein-T_3 complex formed *in vitro* seemed to be entirely similar to that formed *in vivo*, in that it was extracted by 0.4 M KCl, thermolabile at 37° C or higher temperatures, destroyed by pronase, protected by dithiothreitol, destroyed by incubation with PCMB, and moved anodally on electrophoresis.

We found that the nuclear T_4 binding protein-T_3 complex prepared *in vivo* dissociated with a half time of approximately 95 minutes during *in vitro* incubation. This suggested that a significant proportion of the endogenous complex could dissociate during incubation, and that binding could occur through exchange of added T_3 with the endogenous complex, or by addition of T_3 to empty nuclear binding sites. One of the most important conclusions of these studies was that T_3 apparently bound directly to the nuclear complex without mediation of a cytosol protein, in sharp contrast to the systems previously described for binding of estrogen, progesterone, and corticoids with nuclear receptor proteins. Further T_3 analogs such as Triac were found to bind with increased avidity in comparison to T_3, and the relatively inactive dextro-isomer of T_3 was bound as actively as L-T_3 (Figure 1). Thus, factors other than direct binding affinity to the nuclear receptors must be involved in determining the relative biological potency of hormone analogs.

Similar studies have been reported from several laboratories.

Table 3. BINDING OF T_3 TO NUCLEAR RECEPTORS MEASURED *IN VITRO*

Tissue source	Incubation conditions	Capacity			Authors
		$Kd \times 10^{-10}M$	fmoles/ 100 µg DNA	ng/gm liver	
Rat liver nuclei	SMT, pH 7.85 + 5 mM DTT SMCT, pH 7.4	5 15	53 90	.5 1.2	DeGroot & Torresani, '75 DeGroot & Torresani, '75
Rat liver nuclei	SMT, pH 7.0	17			Koerner, Surks, & Oppenheimer, '74
Rat liver nuclei	SMT, pH 7.0	17	60	85	Surks, Koerner, & Oppenheimer, '75
Rat liver nuclei	SMT, pH 7.85 + 5 mM DTT	2.1	100		Samuels & Tsai, '73
GH₁ cells	Hams F-10 Media	.3	100		and
GH₁ nuclei	SMT, pH 7.85 + 5 mM DTT	1.65	104		Samuels & Tsai, '74
Rat liver nuclei	SMT, pH 7.6, 1 mM DTT, + 5% glycerol, 1 mM EDTA	1.9	100		Spindler, MacLeod, Ring, & Baxter, '75
Human lymphocytes	Hams F-10	.3	4		Tsai & Samuels, '74

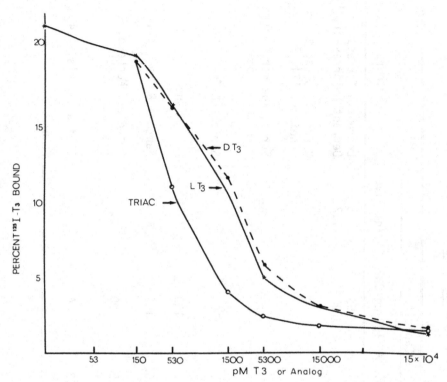

Figure 1.   *Inhibition of T₃ binding by hormone analogues. Nuclei*
prepared in standard manner in SMT-pH 7.85 were incu-
bated in triplicate in 1 ml containing 150 μg DNA, 5 mM
DTT, and 15 pM ¹²⁵I-T₃.   Unlabeled L-T₃, D-T₃, and tri-
iodothyroacetic acid were added to produce the indicated
concentrations.   The ordinate represents percent nuclear
binding of ¹²⁵I-T₃ after 135 min at 20° C.

Koerner *et al.* (1974) reported *in vitro* binding of nuclei obtained
from rats, prepared through sucrose gradient and incubated in .32
M sucrose, 3 mM magnesium chloride, and .02 M Tris at pH 7 in .03%
human albumin.

Binding of T_3 to receptors in rat liver nuclei was studied in
an *in vitro* system by Surks, Koerner, and Oppenheimer (1975). They
found that equilibrium binding occurred in 30 min at 37° C in their
system at pH 7.0, and was unaffected by the addition of inhibitors
of oxidative-phosphorylation. T_3 dissociated from nuclei *in vitro*

with a half time of 0.058^{-1} min. The Ka for T_3 was $0.06 \times 10^{10} M^{-1}$ and binding capacity was 0.85 ng/g liver. The T_3 bound to nuclear receptor sites could be extracted with 0.4 M KCl and moved through Sephadex G-100 columns as a molecule with a molecular size of approximately 60,000 daltons. Addition of cytosol to the system did not alter the affinity constant or binding capacity of the nuclear sites, indicating that cytosol proteins were not required for the binding activity. Nuclei from normal and thyroidectomized animals had similar affinity constants and binding capacity.

Samuels and Tsai (1974) reported similar studies comparing *in vitro* binding of rat liver nuclei and GH-1 cells or nuclei. The affinity constants and binding capacities are indicated in Table 3. Samuels indicated that the rat liver nuclei have binding sites for approximately 7,800 molecules per nucleus, and that the nuclei were about 20% saturated at normal serum T_3 levels. He estimated that 75% of endogenously bound nonradioactive T_3 would dissociate during incubation and, thus, that 95% of total nuclear binding sites for T_3 could be identified in the *in vitro* system.

Spindler, MacLeod, Ring, and Baxter (1975) found a Kd for T_3 in rat liver nuclei *in vitro* of 1.9×10^{-10} M and binding capacity of 100 fmoles/100 µg DNA. Their studies were conducted on Triton-washed nuclei at pH 7.6 in 5% glycerol. Hypothyroid and euthyroid rat liver nuclei had similar binding affinities and capacity. Similar capacity of T_3 binding per mg of DNA was found when nuclei and chromatin prepared from nuclei were studied in parallel experiments.

Samuels and Tsai (1973) studied binding of T_3 *in vitro* to GH-1 cells and nuclei derived from these cells. The dissociation constant in nuclei was 0.3×10^{-10} M, and binding capacity was 65 fmoles/100 µg DNA. The Kd for T_4 was approximately nine times larger. T_4 competitively inhibited the binding of T_3 to the receptors. In this system, the estimated free hormone concentration that produced half-maximal increase in the rate of cell growth and glucose utilization was 8×10^{-9} M, which is somewhat less than the concentration producing half-maximal saturation of the binding sites. Prior incubation of cells, with nonradioactive T_3, at 10^{-12} to 10^{-9} M, augmented capacity of binding when the nuclei were subsequently incubated *in vitro* with T_3. This suggested to Samuels and Tsai that binding sites were trasferred from cytosol to nucleus along with T_3. This is the only report so far suggesting a possible enhancing effect of hormone on nuclear binding capacity, or that cytosol proteins transfer T_3 to the nucleus.

The ability of lymphocytes to bind T_3 during *in vitro* incubations was studied first by Tsai and Samuels (1974), who found a Kd of 0.3×10^{-10}, and a capacity of 4 fmoles/100 µg DNA, which is 5% to 10% of the capacity of other tissues.

Binding of T_3 _in vitro_ to Solubilized Nuclear
Triiodothyronine Protein

Since the protein receptors for T_3 could be extracted from
nuclear preparations with 0.4 M KCl or other high salt-containing
solutions, it became possible to test the ability of T_3 to bind directly to these proteins _in vitro_. Torresani and DeGroot (1975)
reported _in vitro_ studies using nuclear T_4 binding protein preparations made with KMP or Tris-glycine buffer at pH 8.5 with 1 mM
$MgCl_2$ and 0.4 M KCl (TGKM). _In vivo_ labelled nuclear T_4 binding
protein-T_3 complex was about 45% extracted in KMP at pH 7.4 and 74%
was extracted in TGKM. Both increasing salt concentration and
increasing pH were associated with greater extraction of nuclear
proteins. Binding of T_3 to the macromolecular complex was studied
by incubation at 20° C for three hours, by which time maximal binding had occurred. The complex formed was thermolabile, destroyed
by incubation with PCMB, retained T_3 when incubated with Dowex 1X8,
200-400 mesh anion exchange resin for five minutes, and moved anodally as a broad band during polyacrylamide gel electrophoresis.
Nuclear proteins, held at 0° C for several days, lost their ability
to bind T_3, but this could be restored by treatment with 5 mM dithiothreitol. Concentrations of 1-10 mM dithiothreitol enhanced
specific binding of T_3. Optimum pH for binding was between 7.8 and
8.5. Manganese ion at 5 mM concentration inhibited binding, and
EDTA at up to 2 mM mildly reduced binding. Calcium at 1 mM slightly activated binding, and then became inhibitory at 5 mM. Optimum
magnesium concentration was approximately 2.5 mM. RNAse and DNAse
did not alter binding. The Kd for T_3 was approximately 5×10^{-10}
when studied in KMP, and slightly higher when studied in TGKM buffer at pH 8.5 (Table 4). The Ka was enhanced if dithiothreitol
was present in the incubation medium. Binding capacity was about
1 ng/g liver and the binding sites were to some degree nonspecific,
with Triac binding more avidly, D-T_3 essentially equally, and L-T_4
and D-T_4 less avidly than T_3 itself.

Samuels, Tsai, and Casanova (1974) studied the binding of T_3
and T_4 _in vitro_ to KCl extracts of rat liver nuclei and GH-1 and
found Kd of 1.6×10^{-10} for the liver preparation and 1.8×10^{-10}
for the GH-1 nuclei. In contrast, cytosol binding proteins had
considerably less affinity for T_3 and more for T_4.

Thomopoulos, Dastugue, and Defer (1974) studied binding of T_3
in vitro to nonhistone proteins, extracted from rat liver nuclei
and partially purified, in an incubation mixture containing 0.4 M
NaCl, EDTA, MSH at pH 7.5 and the Kd for T_3 was 16×10^{-10}.

Kubica, Nauman, Witkowska, and Nauman (1975) recently reported that T_3 binds to two separate proteins in rat liver nuclear
preparations. These can be separated by chromatography. There is
a time-dependent displacement of T_3 from one to the other during
the several hours after administration of hormone to the animals.

Table 4. BINDING OF T_3 TO NUCLEAR T_4 BINDING PROTEINS IN VITRO

Tissue source	Incubation conditions	Capacity			Authors
		Kd x 10⁻¹⁰M	pmols/mg pr	ng/g liver	
Liver nuclei:					
KMP extract	KMP, 5mM DTT, 20°C	5	.49	.87	Torresani & DeGoot, '75
TGKM extract	TGKM	1.25	.46	.78	
Rat liver nuclei:					
KCl extract	SMT + .25 M KCl + 5 mM DTT, 25°C + 2 mM EDTA	1.6	.29		Samuels & Tsai, '74 Samuels, Tsai, & Casanova, '74
GH₁ nuclei:					
KCl extract	SMT + .25 M KCl + 5 mM DTT, 25°C + 2mM EDTA				Samuels, Tsai, Casanova & Stanley, '74
Rat Liver nu-cleoprotein	pH 7.5, 0.4 M NaCl, 1 mM EDTA, 1 mM MSH	16	1		Thomopoulos, Dastugue & Defer, '74

Relative Binding Affinity of T_3, T_4, and Analogs for Nuclear T_4
Binding Proteins

The ability of various analogs to compete with T_3 for binding
to receptors *in vivo* or *in vitro* has been studied in several laboratories. The results are given in Table 5. In general, D-T_4 competes *in vitro* with about one-half to equal efficiency of L-T_3,
whereas L-T_4 is approximately one-tenth and D-T_4 about 1/20th as
avidly bound as L-T_3. Reverse-T_3 is reported to have less than
1/1000th the affinity of T_3 itself. Triac, in a variety of experiments, has been found to have increased affinity when studied *in
vitro*, but according to Oppenheimer, not when studied *in vivo*.
L-T_2, thyronine, and iodotyrosines do not compete for binding with
T_3. There are a few important differences between the observations
made in various laboratories. One striking discrepancy is the dissociation between the effectiveness of Triac *in vivo* and *in vitro*.
There is also an unaccountable difference in the apparent affinity
of D-T_3 for solubilized receptors when one compares the work of
Torresani and DeGroot (1975) and Koerner *et al.* (1974) to that from
Samuels and Tsai (1974a), who found *in vitro* that D-T_3 possessed
only 10% of the binding activity of L-T_3.

Koerner, Schwartz, Surks, Oppenheimer, and Jorgensen (1975)
have recently studied the binding affinities of a wide spectrum of
thyroid hormone analogs, and found good agreement between nuclear
binding and biologic activity. Binding is greater for 3' mono-
than for 3', 5' di-substituted analogs. A 4'-OH group is needed.
Halogen-free analogs have low activity.

Cytosol Binding Proteins

Proteins that bind T_3 and other forms of thyroid hormone are
also present in the cell cytosol and these have been studied in a
number of laboratories (Table 5). Hocman (1973) studied the cytosol
fraction by chromatography through Sephadex. Dillman, Surks, and
Oppenheimer (1974) found two sets of T_3-binding proteins in cytosol,
one with high capacity and the other with low capacity. The limited
capacity, high affinity sites had a binding equilibrium constant of
$4.3 \times 10^7 M^{-1}$ and a binding capacity of $5.3 \times 10^{-7}M$. Similar binding
proteins were found in kidney cytosol. Thyroxine also bound to this
protein, as did all of the T_3 analogs studied. The association
constant of the cytosol T_3 binding site was only about 0.5% that of
the nuclear binding protein. These authors estimated that, at
plasma T_3 concentrations in rats of 0.83 ng/ml, and with liver to
plasma T_3 ratios of 8, that approximately 30% of the cellular T_3
would be in the cytosol and that 1% of the cytosol T_3 binding sites
would be occupied. This is in contrast to an estimate of 70% nuclear binding site occupancy by T_3 in rats by the same laboratory.
The binding protein in liver appeared to bind T_4 with one-third the
affinity of T_3, and Triac with one-sixth the affinity.

Table 5. RELATIVE RECEPTOR AFFINITY OF T_3 AND ANALOGS

	Oppenheimer, Schwartz, Dillman, & Surks, '73 in vivo, liver	DeGroot & Torresani '75 in vitro, nuclei	Torresani & DeGroot, '75	Koerner, Surks, & Oppenheimer, '74	Samuels & Tsai, '74
	nuclei in vivo	nuclei in vitro	NTBP in vitro	nuclei in vitro	NTBP in vitro
L-T_3	1	1	1	1	1
L-T_4	.1	.25	.1	.11	.08
D-T_3	--	1	.5-.7	.61	.12
D-T_4	--	.08	.04	--	.017
r-T_3	0	--	--	.001	.0025
Triac	1	4	9	1.64	--
Tetrac	0.05	--	--	.16	--
Isopropyl T_2	1.0	--	--	1.04	--
L-T_2	--	--	--	--	.0036
Thyronine	--	--	--	--	.0023
MIT	0	±0	0	0	--
DIT	0	±0	0	0	--

Sterling, Saldanha, Brenner, and Milch (1974) have reported electrophoretic studies of rat liver cytosol binding proteins, and indicated that two T_4 binding proteins are present which appear to be different from thyroid binding globulin of rat serum and at least one protein is present which selectively binds T_3.

Davis, Handwerger, and Glaser (1974) found that rat liver and kidney cytosol proteins, with a molecular weight of approximately 70,000, behaved as specific T_4 binding proteins. Two classes of binding sites on the cytosol proteins were found for T_4, and one for T_3 with a Ka of $2.3 \times 10^7 M^{-1}$. Either hormone was displaced by the other. $D-T_4$, tetraiodothyroacetic acid (Tetrac), and tetra-chlorothyronine competed with T_4 for binding sites on these proteins.

Physiologic Alterations in Nuclear T_4 Binding Protein Capacity or Affinity

The effects of various physiological alterations on nuclear T_4 binding protein have been studied in several laboratories. According to Samuels and Tsai, exposure of GH-1 cells to T_3 *in vitro* increased the nuclear binding capacity. This is in contrast to other reports, in which binding affinity and capacity are found to be similar in hypothyroid and normal animals, or animals given excessive loads of T_3 *in vivo* prior to preparation of the nuclei (Table 6). We have studied the effect of injections of estrogen, androgen, and glucocorticoids on binding affinity and capacity of nuclear binding sites in immature female rats and found no significant effects of these hormones on T_3 binding.

Table 6.   *RELATION OF Ka AND CAPACITY FOR T_3 TO THYROID STATUS*

Animals	Nuclear T_3 content	Ka x $10^{10} M^{-1}$	Capacity pg/g	Capacity pg/100 µg DNA
Normal	± 600 pg/g	.075 ± .05	297 ± 35	47 ± 17
Hypothyroid	10 pg/g	.1 ± .04	239 ± 40	31 ± 14
Hypothyroid + T_3	200-800 pg/g	.094 ± .04	224 ± 70	29 ± 8

Binding affinity and capacity was evaluated *in vitro* using preparations of nuclei from normal rats, thyroidectomized rats, or hypothyroid animals given T_3 prior to sacrifice. There were no significant differences between the groups (DeGroot and Torresani, 1975).

An increase in binding capacity for T_3 in tadpole tail nuclei occurs during metamorphosis, as reported by Yoshizato and Frieden (1975). They found an increase from 1,300 to 2,400 binding sites per cell nucleus, with possible but uncertain alteration in the apparent dissociation constant. These authors suggest that the increase in hormone sensitivity of tail tissue during metamorphosis may be a result of the increase in nuclear binding capacity, rather than an increase in the affinity constant. It is also possible that the increasing supply of T_4 in the animals during metamorphosis increases the nuclear receptors.

We have found an age-dependent increase in nuclear T_3 binding capacity in rats, with capacities of around 10 pg/100 μg DNA in immature rats at one to ten days of life, increasing to 50 pg/100 μg DNA in the mature animals.

Mechanism of T_3 Transport to Nuclei

The exact mechanism of uptake of T_3 from serum and transport to the nucleus remains uncertain. There is no evidence for active transport of T_3 into the cells, and no evidence that T_3 moves into cells in conjunction with serum binding proteins. It is believed that free T_3 diffuses from serum into cell cytosol. Presumably T_3 is in equilibrium with the set of binding proteins present in cytosol, and a free T_3 concentration roughly similar to that present in the serum prevails in cytosol. Possibly there is, in fact, a gradient from cytosol to serum, since T_4 is metabolized in cells by mono-deiodination to produce T_3. There is so far no evidence that T_3 moves into the nucleus attached to a protein. Rather, it appears that free T_3 diffuses into the nucleus and binds to the nuclear receptor proteins. Thus, it may be presumed that free T_3 content of the nucleus is about the same as in cytosol.

Function of the Nuclear T_4 Binding Protein-T_3 Complex

All authors start with the presumption that T_3 acts in the nucleus to alter DNA transcription in some way, leading to formation of new ribosomal or messenger RNA, and ultimately new protein synthesis. As indicated earlier, Tata reported in 1966 that the first observable effect of T_3 administered to hypothyroid rats was to alter the function of the low salt-magnesium-dependent RNA polymerase believed to form ribosomal RNA. Binding of T_3 to histones was reported. We have found that the nuclear T_4 binding protein-T_3 complex binds to chromatin, and that binding is inhibited by high salt concentrations. MacLeod and Baxter (1975) have, likewise, reported that this complex (isolated from rat liver) binds to purified DNA, whereas free T_3 and plasma proteins do not associate with DNA. Binding was observed at 0.15 M KCl. Charles, Ryffel, Obinata, McCarthy,

and Baxter (1975) have studied the association of the complex with
chromatin. Chromatin was prepared from rat liver nuclei which had
been incubated with T_3 *in vitro*. Nuclei were washed in several
buffer systems and chromatin was sheared in a French pressure cell.
Chromatin was then separated by sucrose gradient velocity sedimentation. T_3 receptor complexes were distributed throughout the
chromatin fractions, but were enriched in the slowly sedimenting
fractions which contain most of the template capacity for RNA synthesis and most of the endogenous RNA polymerase activity. When
chromatin-associated nuclear T_4 binding protein-T_3 complex was
treated with formaldehyde, the receptor T_3 complex remained with
the chromatin. This evidence is taken to suggest a close association of the complex with chromatin, and an association with the
portions of the chromatin more active in template activity. Tsai
and Samuels (1974) and Samuels *et al*. (1973) studied the effect of
thyroid hormone added *in vitro* to cultured GH-1 cells. T_3 caused
a three-fold increase in the rate of growth of the cultured GH-1
cells, an increased rate of growth hormone secretion and a decrease in prolactin secretion. TRH stimulation of prolactin secretion was inhibited. T_3 at 3×10^{-11} M free hormone concentration produced half-maximal inhibition of prolactin secretion.

Perhaps the most dramatic reports of T_4 or T_3 action on nuclei
come from studies of Kim and Cohen (1966). The administration of
T_4 to tadpoles for 11 days led to both an increase in the activity
of RNA polymerases and an increased template function of the tadpole chromatin. Chromatin deproteinized by cesium chloride did
not show the difference in template efficiency, indicating that
alterations in the chromatin-associated proteins were responsible
for the differences in template activity.

Sterling and Milch (1975) have reported the presence of specific binding sites for T_3 in rat liver mitochondria. They indicate that the Ka is approximately 2.7×10^{10} M^{-1}, which is considerably higher than that reported for nuclei. It has been estimated
that such binding sites would presumably hold no more than one or
two molecules of T_3 per cell mitochondrion. Nevertheless, the observation suggests that there may be separate binding sites in nuclei and mitochondria.

Dillman, Schwartz, Silva, Surks, and Oppenheimer (1975) have
suggested that T_3 causes an "imprint" with a long half-life which
is involved in the expression of the metabolic action of thyroid
hormone. When 3 µg of T_3 was given per 100 g body weight to hypothyroid rats, a 3- to 4-fold increase in mitochondrial α-glycero-
phosphate dehydrogenase occurred at 24 hours. α-amanitin given at
zero and eight hours blocked this response. Three days after administration of T_3 and α-amanitin, the α-glycerophosphate dehydrogenase activity of the α-amanitin treated animals had recovered
nearly to normal. They suggest T_3 caused an "imprint" which subse-

quently induced an increase in mRNA formation, after the effect of
α-amanitin was dissipated.

Samuels and Tsai (1975) found that actinomycin D inhibited
the augmented production of growth hormone occurring after exposure
of his GH-1 cell line to free T_3 at 1 x 10^{-10} M *in vitro*. Exposure
of the cell line to actinomycin D, 20 hours after incubation with
T_3, produced a slow fall-off in growth hormone production. They
believe that induction of growth hormone production correlates
well with nuclear receptor occupancy, and has a requirement for
RNA synthesis.

Silva, Schwartz, Surks, and Oppenheimer (1975) have reported
that there is close correlation between the stimulation of α-gly-
cerophosphate dehydrogenase activity in hypothyroid rat liver and
the occupancy of receptor sites by T_3. Doses of 20-5,000 μg/100 g
body weight of T_3 were given to rats. It was found that any dose
which saturated more than 95% of the nuclear sites led to maximal
T_3 induced enzyme level at that time. When these sites became de-
saturated, enzyme activity fell rapidly.

Characteristics of Binding of the Nuclear T_4 Binding Protein-T_3 Complex to Chromatin

We have studied binding of liver nuclear T_4 binding protein-
T_3 complex to chromatin under a number of conditions (DeGroot,
Hill, Seo, and Bernal, 1975). The complex was prepared by KCl extraction of liver nuclei labelled with ^{125}I-T_3 *in vivo*. Chromatin
was prepared from rat heart, kidney, spleen, brain, and testis.
Binding was found to be optimal at 0° C over a period of two hours.
More rapid binding occurred at elevated temperatures, but there was
apparent loss of binding activity during incubation apparently due
to degradation of the complex. Binding of the liver receptor complex to chromatin from any of these six tissues was inhibited as
KCl concentration was raised (Figure 2). Most studies were conducted at 0.065 M KCl. Specific binding was considered to be that
occurring in the presence of chromatin as compared to its absence,
or the level of binding occurring with low KCl concentrations
(0.065 M), in contrast to that occurring in high KCl (0.4 M) concentrations. Uptake of the T_3-protein receptor complex was greatest by heart chromatin and declined in the order of heart, testis,
liver, spleen, and brain. While binding of the liver T_3 receptor
complex to heart chromatin was significantly greater than that occurring in brain chromatin, the differences between binding activity in the T_3-responsive tissues (heart, kidney, and liver) was
little higher than that in the tissues assumed to be T_3-nonrespon-
sive (Table 6).

To look at saturability of the binding process, constant

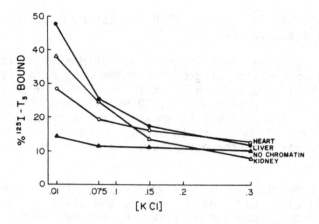

Figure 2. *KCl sensitive binding of nuclear T_4 binding protein to chromatin. ^{125}I-T labelled nuclear T_3 binding protein-T_3 complex from liver nuclei was incubated with chromatin from heart, liver, or kidney for two hours at $0°$ C. Nuclear T_4 binding protein-T_3 complex rebinds to chromatin at low, but not high, KCl concentrations.*

amounts of liver chromatin were incubated with a constant amount of ^{125}I-T_3 *in vivo* labelled nuclear T_4 binding protein-T_3 complex, and increasing amounts of unlabelled complex. It was possible to add up to 16-fold greater amounts of unlabelled protein than that present as the labelled species. No evidence of saturability of the binding sites was detected when liver nuclear receptor proteins were reacted under these conditions with chromatin from any of the six tissues. These studies suggest that, at least under the conditions of the experiments, the binding of the receptor protein-T_3 complex to chromatin is not a tissue specific process, and is not limited by available receptor sites. Although this complex may be the intracellular messenger which ultimately promotes responsiveness to thyroid hormone, its binding to tissue chromatins is of a nonsaturable, high capacity, and relatively nonspecific variety. Capacity for binding of the complex does not seem to correlate with responsiveness of the tissues to hormone. Therefore, we may deduce that the controlling factor in the responsiveness of tissues to T_3 is the concentration of and saturation of the nuclear receptor for the nuclear T_4 binding protein, rather than saturation of chromatin acceptor sites for the complex. Nuclear T_4 binding protein concentration has been found to be low in T_3-nonresponsive tissues such as testis, spleen, and brain, in contrast to the concentrations in responsive tissues.

The data presented allow a hypothetical formulation of the process of T_3 induction of a metabolic response in tissues. Presumably, free T_3 present in serum migrates into cells and is in equilibrium with T_3 bound to cytosol-binding proteins and the free T_3 generated in the cell by monodeiodination of T_4. The cytosol unbound T_3 also diffuses into the nucleus, where it binds to nuclear T_4 binding protein, which may be free or bound to chromatin. The complex is then bound to chromatin and initiates another metabolic step, the nature of which is yet unknown. Evidence suggests that it may be induction of RNA polymerase activity, with augmented mRNA and rRNA synthesis, and ultimately increased protein synthesis. The T_3 receptor sites seem to be relatively specific, saturable, and have a binding affinity for thyroid hormone analogs which roughly parallels their metabolic activity when administered to animals. The Kd of the binding sites observed in whole cells approximates the free level of hormone in serum (ca 10^{-11} M), but it must be admitted that the Kd observed for isolated nuclei or isolated receptor protein is an order of magnitude higher. This may be an artifact of the conditions under which the receptor protein affinity is measured when nuclei or solubilized receptors are studied, in contrast to whole cells such as lymphocytes or GH-1 cells. Further, the Kd of the sites found for GH-1 cells approximates the level of free T_3 which is found to stimulate growth of these cells in culture. Thus, there is some evidence for the importance of the nuclear receptors, although it must be stated that the final proof of their preeminence in the metabolic response to thyroid hormone is lacking, unless one is willing to give strong weight to the clinical studies to be described below.

Clinical Studies on T_3 Nuclear Receptors

We believe we can present data from clinical studies indicating that there is some biologic relevance of the binding proteins. We are fortunate in having at our disposal a sibship reported in two previous publications which appears to have an inherited resistance to thyroid hormone action (Refetoff, DeGroot, Benard, and DeWind, 1972; Refetoff, DeWind, and DeGroot, 1967). These three children in one sibship have high circulating levels of free T_3-- goiter, stippled epiphyses, deaf-mutism, and growth retardation. Hyperphysiologic levels of hormone induced metabolic evidence of hormone activity. We have studied in these children the response to thyroid releasing hormone (TRH) and find that the pituitaries secrete thyroid stimulating hormone (TSH) in response to TRH, even when the endogenous T_3 level is 300 ng/dl. The administration of 100 μg T_3/day further augments T_3 levels in serum and, if anything, TRH responsiveness is enhanced. Quite clearly, the pituitary of these children shares in the nonresponsiveness or partial responsiveness to thyroid hormone. Prednisone, which is known to nonspecificially inhibit TRH secretion or pituitary responsiveness to TRH, inhibited the response in these children as well.

We examined in more detail the binding sites for T_3 in the nu-

clei of these children by studying the function of lymphocytes using
methods previously reported by Tsai and Samuels (1974). Lymphocytes of nine normal adults were found to have a Kd for T_3 of 2.5 x
10^{-10}M and capacity 4.5 fmoles/100 μg DNA, with average plasma
T_3 levels of 135 ng/dl. Younger children had higher binding
affinities and slightly lower capacities. In one child of the T_3
resistant sibship, duplicate studies showed that binding affinity
was approximately 1/10th that of normal, and capacity 10 fmoles
T_3/100 μg DNA (Bernal, DeGroot, Refetoff, Fang, and Barsano, 1975).
It is possible that the Kd, in fact, represents the absence of any
specific binding sites, since it would be difficult to determine
that the very low affinity reflects other than nonspecific binding.
We further examined the function of the binding sites in these
children by separating the *in vivo*-labelled nuclei and extracting
the *in vitro*-labelled nuclear T_4 binding protein-T_3 complex with
KCl. We could recover about 50% of the isotope in the extract,
and of this about one-half behaved as a protein-bound form of T_3.
However, when this labelled complex was incubated with human lymphocyte nuclear chromatin, minimal binding occurred. In contrast,
a similar binding protein-T_3 complex obtained from normal human
lymphocyte nuclei bound to chromatin in a KCl sensitive manner.
Whether this represents an abnormality of the binding protein or a
total lack of the normal protein is unknown. We also have not completed the experiments which will rule out any possible deficiency
in the chromatin. Thus, children with a syndrome of marked, inherited resistance to thyroid hormone have minimal or absent nuclear binding sites, and the binding material present does behave
in an abnormal way. This rather strongly points to an importance
for the binding sites in a physiologic response of the human or
experimental animal to the metabolic stimulatory effects of thyroid
hormone.

REFERENCES

Bernal, J., DeGroot, L.J., Refetoff, S., Fang, V.S., and Barsano,
    C. (1975) Absent nuclear thyroid hormone receptors and fail-
    ure of T_3-induced TRH suppression in the syndrome of peripher-
    al resistance to thyroid hormone. *Excerpta Medica* 361:66.
Blobel, G. and Potter, V.R. (1966) Nuclei from rat liver: Isola-
    tion method that combines purity with high yield. *Science*
    154:1662-1665.
Charles, M.A., Ryffel, G.U., Obinata, M., McCarthy, B.J., and
    Baxter, J.D. (1975) Nuclear receptors for thyroid hormone:
    Evidence for nonrandom distribution within chromatin. *Proc.
    Nat'l. Acad. Sci.* 72:1787-1791.
Davis, P.J., Handwerger, B.S., and Glaser, F. (1974) Physical
    properties of a dog liver and kidney cytosol protein that
    binds thyroid hormone. *J. Biol. Chem.* 249:6208-6217.
DeGroot, L.J., Hill, L., Seo, H., and Bernal, J. (1975) Factors
    influencing T_3 binding to nuclear protein and chromatin.
    Excerpta Medica 361:66-67.

DeGroot, L.J., Refetoff, S., Strausser, J., and Barsano, C. (1974)
    Nuclear triiodothyronine-binding protein: Partial character-
    ization and binding to chromatin. *Proc. Nat'l. Acad. Sci.*
    71:4042-4046.
DeGroot, L.J. and Strausser, J.L. (1974) Binding of T₃ in rat
    liver nuclei. *Endocrinology* 95:74-83.
DeGroot, L.J. and Torresani, J. (1975) Triiodothyronine binding
    to isolated liver cell nuclei. *Endocrinology* 96:375-369.
Dillman, W., Schwartz, H.L., Silva, E., Surks, M.I., and Oppen-
    heimer, J.H. (1975) Evidence for the role of RNA polymerase
    II and a long-lived triiodothyronine (T₃) 'imprint' in the
    expression of thyroid hormone action. *Excerpta Medica* 361:
    83-84.
Dillman, W., Surks, M.I., and Oppenheimer, J.H. (1974) Quantita-
    tive aspects of iodothyronine binding by cytosol proteins of
    rat liver and kidney. *Endocrinology* 95:492-498.
Griswold, M.D., Fischer, M.S., and Cohen, P.P. (1972) Temperature-
    dependent intracellular distribution of thyroxine in amphib-
    ian liver. *Proc. Nat'l. Acad. Sci.* 69:1486-1489.
Hocman, G. (1973) Gel filtration of thyroxine-binding proteins:
    Group separation of soluble proteins of rat liver on Sephadex
    gels. *Int. J. Biochim.* 4:531-535.
Kim, K.H. and Cohen, P.P. (1966) Modification of tadpole liver
    chromatin by thyroxine treatment. *Biochemistry* 55:1251-1255.
Koerner, D., Schwartz, H.L., Surks, M.I., Oppenheimer, J.H., and
    Jorgensen, E.C. (1975) Binding of selected iodothyronine
    analogs to receptor sites of isolated rat hepatic nuclei.
    High correlation between structural requirements for nuclear
    binding and biological activity. *J. Biol. Chem.* 250:6417-
    6423.
Koerner, D., Surks, M.I., and Oppenheimer, J.H. (1974) *In vitro*
    demonstration of specific triiodothyronine binding sites in
    rat liver nuclei. *J. Clin. Endocrinol. Metab.* 38:706-709.
Kubica, A., Nauman, A., Witkowska, E., and Nauman, J. (1975) Bind-
    ing of T₃ in liver nuclei: Time-dependent displacement of T₃
    between two nuclear binding proteins. *Excerpta Medica* 361:
    67-68.
MacLeod, K.M. and Baxter, J.D. (1975) DNA binding of thyroid hor-
    mone receptors. *Biophys. Res. Comm.* 62:577-583.
Oppenheimer, J.H., Koerner, D., Schwartz, H.L., and Surks, M.I.
    (1972) Specific nuclear triiodothyronine binding sites in
    rat liver and kidney. *J. Clin. Endocrinol. Metab.* 35:330-
    333.
Oppenheimer, J.H., Schwartz, H.L., Dillman, W., and Surks, M.I.
    (1973) Effect of thyroid hormone analogs on the displacement
    of ¹²⁵I-L-triiodothyronine from hepatic and heart nuclei *in
    vivo*: Possible relationship to hormonal activity. *Biochem.
    Biophys. Res. Comm.* 55:544-550.
Oppenheimer, J.H., Schwartz, H.L., Koerner, D., and Surks, M.I.

(1974) Nuclear-cytoplasmic interrelation, binding constants, and cross-reactivity with L-thyroxine. *J. Clin. Invest.* 53: 768-777.

Oppenheimer, J.H., Schwartz, H.L., and Surks, M.I. (1974) Tissue differences in the concentration of triiodothyronine nuclear binding sites in the rat: Liver, kidney, pituitary, heart, brain, spleen, and testis. *Endocrinology* 95:897-903.

Refetoff, S., DeGroot, L.J., Benard, B., and DeWind, L.T. (1972) Studies of a sibship with apparent hereditary resistance to the intracellular action of thyroid hormone. *Metabolism* 21: 723-756.

Refetoff, S., DeWind, L.T., and DeGroot, L.J. (1967) Familial syndrome combining deaf-mutism, stippled epiphyses, goiter, and abnormally high PBI: Possible target organ refractoriness to thyroid hormone. *J. Clin. Endocrinol. Metab.* 27: 279-294.

Samuels, H.H. and Tsai, J.S. (1975) Induction of growth hormone by triiodothyronine: Evidence for regulation at the nuclear level. *Excerpta Medica* 361:84-85.

Samuels, H.H. and Tsai, J.S. (1974a) *In vitro* association of thyroid hormone and hormal analogs with solubilized nuclear receptors of rat liver and cultured GH_1 cells. Program of the 56th Annual Meeting of the Endocrine Society, Abstract No. 78.

Samuels, H.H. and Tsai, J.S. (1974b) Thyroid hormone action. Demonstration of similar receptors in isolated nuclei of rat liver and cultured GH_1 cells. *J. Clin. Invest.* 53:656-659.

Samuels, H.H. and Tsai, J.S. (1973) Thyroid hormone action in cell culture: Demonstration of nuclear receptors in intact cells and isolated nuclei. *Proc. Nat'l. Acad. Sci.* 70:3488-3492.

Samuels, H.H. Tsai, J.S., and Casanova, J. (1974) Thyroid hormone action: *In vitro* demonstration of putative receptors in isolated nuclei and soluble nuclear extracts. *Science* 184:1188-1191.

Samuels, H.H., Tsai, J.S., Casanova, J., and Stanley, F. (1974) Thyroid hormone action. *In vitro* characterization of solubilized nuclear receptors from rat liver and cultured GH_1 cells. *J. Clin, Invest.* 54:853-865.

Samuels, H.H., Tsai, J.S., and Cintron, R. (1973) Thyroid hormone action: A cell-culture system responsive to physiological concentrations of thyroid hormones. *Science* 181:1253-1256.

Schadlow, A.R., Surks, M.I., Schwartz, H.L., and Oppenheimer, J.H. (1972) Specific triiodothyronine binding sites in the anterior pituitary of the rat. *Science* 176:1252-1254.

Silva, E., Schwartz, H.L., Surks, M.I., and Oppenheimer, J.H. (1975) Relationship of nuclear occupancy by triiodothyronine to hepatic response as inferred from the activity of two hepatic enzymes. Program of the 57th Annual Meeting of the Endocrine Society, Abstract No. 135.

Spindler, B.J., MacLeon, K.M., Ring, J., and Baxter, J.D. (1975)
    Thyroid hormone receptors. Binding characteristics and lack
    of hormonal dependency for nuclear localization. *J. Biol.
    Chem.* 250:4113-4119
Sterling, K. and Milch, P.O. (1975) The mitochondria as a site of
    thyroid hormone action. *Excerpta Medica* 361:68.
Sterling, K., Saldanha, V.F., Brenner, M.A., and Milch, P.O. (1974)
    Cytosol-binding protein of thyroxine and triiodothyronine in
    human and rat kidney tissue. *Nature* 250:661-663.
Surks, M.I., Koerner, D., Dillman, W., and Oppenheimer, J.H. (1973)
    Limited capacity binding sites for L-triiodothyronine in rat
    liver nuclei. Localization to the chromatin and partial char-
    acterization of the L-triiodothyronine-chromatin complex. *J.
    Biol. Chem.* 246:7066-7072.
Surks, M.I., Koerner, D.H., and Oppenheimer, J.H. (1975) *In vitro*
    binding of L-triiodothyronine to receptors in rat liver nu-
    clei. Kinetics of binding, extraction properties, and lack
    of requirement for cytosol proteins. *J. Clin. Invest.* 55:50-
    60.
Tabachnick, M. and Giorgio, N.A. (1966) Interaction of thyroid
    hormone with histone from calf thymus nuclei. *Nature* 212:
    1610-1611.
Tata, J.R., Ernster, L., and Suranyi, E.M. (1962) Interaction be-
    tween thyroid hormones and cellular constituents. *Biochim.
    Biophys. Acta* 60:480-491.
Tata, J.R. and Widnell, C.C. (1966) Ribonucleic acid synthesis
    during the early action of thyroid hormones. *Biochem. J.*
    98:604-620.
Thomopoulos, P., Dastugue, B., and Defer, N. (1974) *In vitro* tri-
    iodothyronine binding to non-histone proteins from rat liver
    nuclei. *Biochem. Biophys. Res. Comm.* 58:499-506.
Torresani, J. and DeGroot, L.J. (1975) Triiodothyronine binding
    to liver nuclear solubilized proteins *in vitro*. *Endocrinology*
    96:1201-1209.
Tsai, J.S. and Samuels, H.H. (1974a) Thyroid hormone action:
    Demonstration of putative nuclear receptors in human lympho-
    cytes. *J. Clin. Endocrinol. Metab.* 38:919-922.
Tsai, J.S. and Samuels, H.H. (1974b) Thyroid hormone action:
    Stimulation of growth hormone and inhibition of prolactin
    secretion in cultured GH$_1$ cells. *Biochem. Biophys. Res. Comm.*
    59:420-428.
Yoshizato, K. and Frieden, E. (1975) Increase in binding capacity
    for triiodothyronine in tadpole tail nuclei during metaphosis.
    Nature 254:705-706.

DISCUSSION FOLLOWING DR. DeGROOT'S TALK

Dr. Feigelson
Do you have any indications as to whether your T_3 protein complex is binding to DNA or protein portions of your chromatin?

Dr. DeGroot
No, we haven't finished those experiments.

Dr. Feigelson
Does it bind to pure DNA?

Dr. DeGroot
It's been reported that the T_3-protein complex binds to pure DNA. I haven't looked at the binding of the complex to pure DNA.

Dr. Hechter
In view of the fact that the nuclear binding proteins do not seem to exhibit stereospecificity, could your findings possibly be due to contamination of the d-form with the l-form?

Dr. DeGroot
The D form has about 5% or 10% of the metabolic activity of the l-form in man and in animals, and its activity is not due to contamination.

Dr. Hechter
Could it be that we are dealing not with the actual receptor but with a device for the storage of bioactive molecules in an organism that has developed fantastic strategies to keep levels of T_3 and T_4 constant? With the hypothalamic-pituitary system and the strongly binding serum proteins keeping concentrations constant, is this another device, this time within the cell, to keep available always the T_3 that is so essential to cell function?

Dr. DeGroot
I have given you what data was available to suggest their importance. I think your question is certainly provocative, and who can say that these are the important binding sites? We've said that those in serum are not and those in cytosol are not, and I can't prove that these in nuclei are the important ones. I have the feeling that T_3 does not work in free solution but must work complexed with some molecule some place, so I presume there are important binding proteins. I think your suggestion is a reasonable one--that these are modulating factors, "buffers," rather than the true receptor, which so far remains elusive. I do think that the NTBP sites are saturable, and I think the fact that they are saturable and their capacity is limited may be adequately put into a control mechanism. I don't think the fact that the binding of the complex to chromatin appears at this time to be nonsaturable

destroys that idea; it just suggests that the response is not
limited by the number of binding proteins which could go on
chromatin. I think perhaps it's better to accept your remark as
a good idea to keep in one's mind rather than try to belabor the
point.

Dr. Hechter
     What is the rate of metabolism of d-thyroxine? Is it differ-
ent from that of 1-thyroxine?

Dr. DeGroot
     I'm afraid I cannot give you the exact data on that. There
have been studies of both rat and man. D-thyroxine is taken up
relatively rapidly by the liver. It is also more rapidly metabolized than LT_3, and it's thought that the rate of metabolism is
only one factor and that there may be other phenomena. I mentioned the difference in binding site affinity. For example, triac is
bound very strongly in serum, and this serum binding may tend to
keep most of the triac out of the cells and away from the nucleus.
But there also may be steps that go on after binding that we don't
understand at all.

Dr. Schrader
     I wonder, Dr. DeGroot, if the chromatin used for your satura-
tion studies was from euthyroid or hypothyroid animals? Maybe the
chromatin used already contains these receptors on the chromatin
units. Did you try extracting the chromatin first?

Dr. DeGroot
     What we have used as chromatin is obviously a matter of defi-
nition. We use Spellsberg's method of preparing the chromatin,
which involves a .35 molar sodium chloride extraction in the first
step and numerous washes. We've used both hypothyroid and normal
chromatin and did not get any difference in binding. (Chromatin
is not a pure substance, let us say, and one just defines a certain preparation.)

Dr. Hagen
     In children with the probable receptor defect, do you think
their T_4 and T_3 turnover is slow? Does this account for the higher serum level? Did you check turnover rates? Presumably, if
there's lack of receptors in the periphery, the metabolism of the
hormones might well be slowed.

Dr. DeGroot
     Their hormone turnover was greatly elevated, with about five
times normal T_3 degradation rates and normal tissue penetration
rates. We did those studies some time ago.

Dr. Prahlad

What controls the level of thyroid hormone receptors? And my second question is: you have mentioned that thyroid hormones may not bind to mitochondria. However, recent studies indicate mitochondrial involvement in thyroid hormone action. Would you comment on that?

Dr. DeGroot

The only variations that I'm aware of in these receptors are the ones I've mentioned. Namely, (1) these children and (2) differences in tissue concentrations which Oppenheimer believes correlate with responsivity, and (3) the neonatal rats that I've mentioned. It has been reported that the concentration of receptors in tadpole tail nuclei goes up during metamorphosis, but to my knowledge those are the only reported variations in content of the binding protein or receptor.

About the effect on mitochondria; Ken Sterling has been a very strong supporter of the idea that mitochondria have receptors for T_3 that are as specific and have as high affinity as nuclei. He presented this data at two meetings. I would say that the majority opinion was that it was surprising data, and that the affinity constants were remarkably high and the quantity bound was remarkably low. Tata's paper in *Nature* just this last month again raises the possibility of mitochondrial receptors, so I don't think it's excluded so far that there are binding sites, or receptors, in other cell components. In our own work we did not find evidence for saturable receptors of the same order of affinity in any part of the cell except the nucleus.

Question

Can one separate the binding of T_3 to the receptors that are involved with regulation of target cell metabolism from the binding of T_3 to enzymes which degrade the hormone?

Dr. DeGroot

Well, I think that you raise a point that's really unanswered by any of the available data. Certainly the nuclei do not appear to be involved in metabolism of T_3. One finds in the nuclei predominantly T_3 during the first few half lives of T_3 disappearance from serum, and not metabolites of T_3. Nuclei incubated *in vitro* with T_3 don't metabolize it, so I think that the nuclei probably are not involved in T_3 metabolism. Whether the receptor pathways and deiodination pathways are branching or sequential, or how they are connected with the deiodinated metabolism of T_3 is quite unknown. Deiodination seems to be mainly a cytosol or microsomal function, and it seems that the nuclei are not involved in deiodination. My theory is that the free T_3 is in equilibrium in the system. There is a reversible equilibrium with some T_3 in serum, some in cytosol, and some in the nucleus, and an equilibrium with-

in each of those compartments with the T_3 bound to the proteins
that have high or low affinity in those compartments. We don't
really know the answer to your question, but I think that these
receptors are separate from the T_3 degradative pathways.

Dr. Siegel
     If I understood one of your slides, it looked to me like
there was a tremendous amount of binding sites in the pituitary
relative to other organs that are very active in terms of their
response to the thyroid hormones, yet we generally don't regard,
I think, the pituitary that way. Do you have any comment about
that?

Dr. DeGroot
     The suggestion is that the concentration of binding sites in
the pituitary is very high. In fact, one can show saturation of
the receptor sites in pituitary using whole tissue homogenates
without even getting out the nuclei, and you cannot do this in the
other tissues. I'm not sure I would agree that the pituitary is
not a highly T_3-responsive tissue; it seems to me it is a very T_3-
responsive tissue. Certainly T_3 rapidly alters things like production of TSH through a protein synthesizing mechanism. Likewise, it inhibits the response to prolactin production, and, more
importantly, stimulates growth hormone secretion in a very sensitive manner. It can be used to calibrate T_3 responsiveness.

Dr. Siegel
     Is pituitary very responsive to thyroid hormone in terms of
the metabolism of the cells; do we know anything about that?

Dr. DeGroot
     Well, it's known, if you go back and look at the paper of
Barker many years ago, that it is a responsive tissue.

STUDIES ON THE GLUCOCORTICOID RECEPTOR AND THE HORMONAL

MODULATION OF THE mRNA FOR TRYPTOPHAN OXYGENASE

Leelavati Ramanarayanan-Murthy, Paul D. Colman, and
Philip Feigelson

Institute of Cancer Research & Department of Biochemistry
College of Physicians and Surgeons of Columbia University
New York, NY 10032

INTRODUCTION

The important role played by steroid hormones in development
and physiological regulation in animals has led investigators over
the past few decades to attempt to unravel and understand the molecular mechanisms involved in the function of steroid hormones.
Several studies have shown that the steroid hormones, including
the glucocorticoid hormone, bind with high affinity to specific
receptor proteins in the target cell cytoplasm. The glucocorticoid-
receptor complex has been shown to undergo an alteration to an
"activated" state which has high affinity for chromosomal sites
within the cell nucleus. This glucocorticoid-receptor interaction
with the genome accompanies, and is presumed to be responsible for,
the cellular responses characteristic of the hormone and its target
tissues. The receptor proteins promise to be useful probes in
understanding genetic control mechanisms and also the organization
and structure of the eukaryotic chromosomes.

Considerable information exists concerning the cellular and
metabolic alterations evoked by glucocorticoid hormones acting upon
responsive tissues. Extensive efforts are now devoted to gaining
an understanding of the molecular processes underlying these hormonally-induced alterations. Over the past few years every possible
control mechanism has been advocated. These include transcriptional
control, translational control, hormone-controlled cytoplasmic, and
nuclear receptors and changes in enzymes and mRNA stabilities. The
recent and ongoing rapid developments in molecular biology have provided interesting concepts and hypotheses concerning gene expression
and its control. Experimental tools that allow direct measurements
of cellular parameters, such as measurement of specific species of

mRNA, have been of great value in these studies.

Most of the models proposed to explain the mechanism of glucocorticoid hormone action, are based on the following postulates:
(1) the hormone enters the target cells; (2) the target tissues
contain receptors; (3) the receptors are located in the cytoplasm
and are translocated into the nucleus when complexed with the hormone; and (4) these events are believed to precede and lead to an
alteration in the pattern of gene expression. Using the biochemical techniques presently available, the first three of these assumptions have been confirmed. All findings to date, with respect
to the glucocorticoid hormones, are compatible with the fourth as-
sumption as well. However, it must be recognized that definitive
insight into any of these processes still remains to be established. Ongoing investigations towards understanding the molecular
mechanisms involved are focused upon the chemical nature of the
cytoplasmic receptor, particularly with respect to its active
sites which interact with the steroid hormone and chromatin; the
chemistry of the changes in the cytoplasmic steroid-receptor complex as it undergoes "activation;" the processes underlying translocation of the activated cytoplasmic receptor into the nucleus;
identification of the specific nuclear sites with which it interacts particularly with respect to the role of the chromosomal proteins and of specific sequences of DNA; a clarification of the
molecular events which subsequently ensue in the nucleus concerning
the specific hormonally-regulated genes; and a description of the
processing of the gene transcript and its ultimate cytoplasmic
translation. In this context, this article reviews the recent
studies conducted in our laboratory, attempting to elucidate the
biochemical processes by which the glucocorticoids regulate the
hepatic enzyme levels.

Glucocorticoid Receptor

It is generally accepted that hormones exert their physiologic
effects after first combining with specific target cell proteins.
In the case of steroids, as originally described for estrogen
(Jensen and Jacobson, 1962), these proteins are soluble cytoplasmic
components of target tissues capable of interacting with high affinity and stereospecificity for the biologically active steroid.
The existence of soluble, intracellular proteins which bind other
steroid hormones (i.e., progesterone, aldosterone, dihydrotestosterone) have since been documented. For reviews see Tomkins,
Gelehrter, Granner, Martin, Samuels, and Thompson (1969); Feldman,
Funder, and Edelman (1972); Jensen and DeSombre (1973); O'Malley
and Means (1974); King and Mainwaring (1974). These intracellular
steroid hormone-binding proteins are now commonly referred to as
"receptors."

Rat liver contains three soluble proteins which bind natural glucocorticoids (Beato and Feigelson, 1972). One of these cytosol proteins is identical with serum transcortin, also known as corticosteroid binding globulin (CBG). Another liver cytosol protein, the "B" protein, also binds the natural glucocorticoids, crossreacts with antibodies prepared to serum transcortin, and is likely to be structurally related to it (Koblinsky, 1973). Like many other serum proteins, transcortin is synthesized in the liver and is released into the plasma (Westphal, 1971). It is not known whether the "B" protein, which is immunologically related to transcortin, is a precursor of or is derived from transcortin or whether it has another biosynthetic origin. Both transcortin and the "B" protein bind naturally-occurring glucocorticoids such as corticosterone and hydrocortisone, but neither binds the synthetic fluorinated glucocorticoids, such as dexamethasone and triamcinolone, compounds which are highly potent glucocorticoids *in vivo*.

There is a third protein present in hepatic cytosol which binds the natural glucocorticoids and also has very high affinity for the synthetic 9α-fluorinated glucocorticoids. Several lines of evidence testify that this third cytoplasmic component, termed the glucocorticoid receptor or G-protein, serves the physiological function of mediating glucocorticoid action. It is believed to be the biologically significant glucocorticoid receptor by virtue of the following four observations:

1. it has specific high affinity saturable binding for natural as well as synthetic biologically active glucocorticoids (Koblinsky, Beato, Kalimi, and Feigelson, 1972);

2. as a steroid-receptor complex it undergoes a time and temperature-dependent "activation" enabling its binding to nuclei, chromatin, and stripped DNA (Kalimi, Colman, and Feigelson, 1975);

3. both *in vivo* and *in vitro* its subcellular translocation from the cytoplasm to the nucleus is a function of its saturation with glucocorticoid (Beato, Kalimi, Beato, and Feigelson, 1974); and

4. time course and steroid dose-response experiments indicate parallel saturation of steroid receptor with hormonal induction of rat liver tryptophan-oxygenase catalytic activity (Beato, Kalimi, and Feigelson, 1972) and specific mRNA level (Schutz, Beato, and Feigelson, 1972, 1973).

Physical and Chemical Properties of the Glucocorticoid Receptor

Unlike transcortin which in sucrose density gradient centrifugation sediments at 4S independently of ionic strength, the hepatic dexamethasone-binding protein sediments in low salt gradients primarily as a 7S complex, which reverts reversibly to the lighter 4S species in the presence of 0.3M NaCl. A similar salt-dependent dissociation is demonstrable by gel-filtration chromatography of the dexamethasone binding protein through Sephadex G-200. A comparable and presumably identical dexamethasone binding protein exists in other glucocorticoid-responsive tissues such as kidney and thymus and to a much lesser extent in spleen, lung, heart, and testis (Beato and Feigelson, 1972).

A summary of the physical characteristics and molecular properties for the three glucocorticoid binding components from rat liver cytosol is presented in Table 1 (Koblinsky et al., 1972).

Table 1. PHYSICAL PARAMETERS OF GLUCOCORTICOID-BINDING PROTEINS OF RAT LIVER CYTOSOL AND SERUM TRANSCORTIN

Physical parameter	Liver transcortin	B protein	Serum transcortin	Receptor protein 0.1μ	Receptor protein 0.3μ
Stokes radius (a)(Å)	29.7	36.7	36.6	45	39
Sedimentation coefficient ($S_{20, w}$)	4.1	4.2	4.2	7.0	4.1
Partial specific volume (v_{20}) (ml/g)	0.729	0.729	0.723		
Molecular weight (Mol wt)x10^{-3}	51.3	64.1	62.6	200	66
Frictional ratio (f/fo)	1.11	1.28	1.29		1.35
Isoelectric point	5.1	4.3			

(Koblinsky et al., 1972)

The sensitivity of transcortin, the B protein, and the receptor to various degradative enzymes is summarized in Table 2. It can be seen that nucleases, lipase, collagenase, hyaluronidase, and neuraminidase do not affect these steroid-binding components, whereas all the proteases tested caused a marked reduction in specific steroid-binding capacities (Koblinsky *et al.*, 1972) thus indicating that the glucocorticoid receptor is a protein with no functional moieties sensitive to these other enzymes.

Table 2. *EFFECTS OF HYDROLYTIC ENZYMES UPON GLUCOCORTICOID-BINDING PROTEINS OF RAT LIVER CYTOSOL*

Enzymatic pretreatment	%[^{3}H] Cortisol bound Transcortin	%[^{3}H] Dexamethasone bound	
		B protein	Receptor
None	100	100	100
Deoxyribonuclease	100	100	110
Ribonuclease	100	100	109
Pronase	3	0.5	43
Papain	83	50	7
Trypsin	14	2	1
Chymotrypsin	8	3	0
Neuraminidase (*V. cholerae*)	92	115	108
Neuraminidase (*Clostridium perfringens*)			85
Hyaluronidase			78
Collagenase	71	100	82
Lipase	103	86	104

(Koblinsky *et al.*, 1972)

Table 3. *THERMODYNAMIC PARAMETERS OF GLUCOCORTICOID BINDING TO*
         RAT LIVER CYTOSOL PROTEINS

Sample	Steroid	$K_a, 0°$ $\times 10^8$	$\Delta G°, 0°$ kcal/mole	$\Delta H°$ kcal/mole	$\Delta S°, 0°$ kcal/mole
G protein	[^{3}H] Dexa-methasone	7.3	-11.0	- 6.1	18.0
Transcortin	[^{3}H] Corti-costerone	30.2	-11.8	-23.7	-43.4
B protein	[^{3}H] Corti-costerone	9.6	-11.2	-19.2	-29.1

(Koblinsky, 1973)

Presented in Table 3 are the equilibrium association constants and derived thermodynamic parameters for the three glucocorticoid binding proteins of rat liver. Furthermore, at all temperatures studied, the binding of cortisol to transcortin and the B protein was accompanied by a negative change in entropy, while binding of dexamethasone to the receptor results in a positive entropy change. This difference in the entropy contribution to the free energy of binding, indicates that the receptor interacts differently with glucocorticoids than do transcortin and the B protein (Koblinsky et al., 1972). It has been previously reported by Westphal (1971) that the binding of cortisol to serum transcortin is accompanied by a negative entropy change, consistent with that observed for hepatic transcortin and the B protein. It is interesting to note, however, that the binding of various steroids to serum albumin demonstrates a positive entropy change similar to that for dexamethasone binding to the receptor. An explanation for this positive entropy change, associated with steroid binding, may be the displacement of relatively ordered protein bound water from the receptor steroid binding site.

Stereospecificity of Steroid Binding to the Receptor

Competition binding experiments employing a wide spectrum of steroid analogs lead to the following conclusions governing stereospecificity of the receptor's binding site for glucocorticoids (Koblinsky, 1973);

1. The planar structure of the α, β unsaturated ketone in the A-ring is essential for steroid binding to all three hepatic cortisol binding components.

2. Aromatization of the A-ring, with loss of the 3-keto moiety and imparting planarity to the A-ring prevents steroid binding to transcortin, the B protein and the receptor. The introduction of a single double bond between C_1 and C_2 in the A-ring, reduces considerably the binding to both transcortin and the B protein while enhancing steroid binding to the receptor. Examples of this kind of substitution are prednisolone and prednisone.

3. Substitutions on the *alpha* side of the steroid decrease, or eliminate binding to transcortin and the B protein while enhancing the affinity of the steroid for the receptor. Such polar groups as 9α-F or 14α-OH inhibit the binding to transcortin; even the insertion of a hydrophobic methyl group into the 6α position decreased the affinity to both transcortin and the B protein. These same substitutions, however, appear to enhance the binding to the receptor.

4. The 17α-OH appears nonessential for the binding to the three hepatic proteins. Its presence on the *alpha* side actually decreases the affinity for all steroids tested including cortisol, 17α-OH progesterone, and cortexolone.

5. The substitution of the 11β-OH function by a ketone group, as with cortisone, interferes with the binding to all three proteins. Complete elimination of the 11-oxyfunction imparts a greater loss in affinity to the receptor protein than to transcortin or the B protein.

6. The α-ketol function in the side chain is more important for the binding of glucocorticoids to the glucocorticoid receptor than it is for the binding to transcortin or the B protein. For example, substitution of the C_{20} keto group with a hydroxyl group or oxidation of the C_{25}-OH to an aldehyde completely eliminates binding to the dexamethasone site of the receptor but still allows considerable binding to transcortin. However, substituting a methyl group for the C_{21} hydroxyl as with 11β-OH progesterone, does not greatly affect its binding to any of the three proteins. Acetylation at C_{21} interferes more markedly with the binding to the receptor protein than with that to transcortin and the B protein. Esterification of the C_{21} hydroxyl with succinate resulting in a charged side chain, still allows binding to transcortin and the B protein while it eliminates binding to the dexamethasone binding site of the receptor.

In summary, the competition analysis reviewed above indicates that the binding of glucocorticoid to transcortin and the B protein most likely involves hydrophobic interaction of the *alpha* side, while the glucocorticoid receptor interacts with the *beta* side of the steroid requiring the 3-Keto, the 11β-OH, and the $C_{20,21}$ side chain (Koblinsky, 1973).

Properties of the Steroid Receptor Complex--Transformation to a Binding Complex

As indicated above, a variety of studies have demonstrated

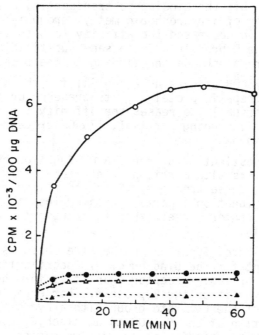

Figure 1. Activation of $[^3H]$ triamcinolone-receptor complex enabling its binding to DNA-cellulose. Each time point represents the extent of binding of $[^3H]$ triamcinolone-receptor complex to DNA-cellulose at 0°. ▲---▲ represents the binding of free steroid alone; ●---● represents binding after cytosol is preincubated with triamcinolone at 0° for 30 minutes, △---△ represents binding after cytosol alone was preincubated at 20° for 30 minutes, then cooled to 0°, and $[^3H]$ triamcinolone was added; 0---0 represents the binding of cytosol-$[^3H]$ triamcinolone preincubated at 20° for 30 minutes (Kalimi et al., 1975).

that the receptor protein of hepatic cytosol has high affinity and stereospecificity to glucocorticoid hormones, both natural and synthetic. The degree of saturation *in vivo* of this cytoplasmic receptor by steroid coincides with its inducing effects upon tryptophan oxygenase and tyrosine aminotransferase (Beato *et al.*, 1972).

The glucocorticoid-receptor complex from hepatoma will bind to free DNA (Baxter, Rousseau, Benson, Garcea, Ito, and Tomkins, 1972). Comparable results with estrogen and aldosterone receptors have demonstrated that a temperature-dependent process was required to convert those steroid-receptor complexes to the form capable of interacting with DNA (Anderson and Liao, 1968; Gorski, Toft, Shyamala, Smith, and Notides, 1968). As depicted in Figure 1 (Kalimi *et al.*, 1975), a similar phenomenon is manifested by the hepatic glucocorticoid-receptor complex. This study indicates that when the receptor-steroid complex is kept at 0°C and allowed to become saturated with triamcinolone, this complex will not bind to DNA at this low temperature. However, if the steroid-receptor complex formed at 0°C is briefly warmed to the higher temperature of 20°C and then recooled to 0°C, it will now bind to DNA-cellulose at 0°C. Controls demonstrate that preheating either the cytosol alone or the steroid alone does not impart the capability to bind to DNA. Thus, at 20°C, an activation or transformation of the steroid-receptor complex occurs, enabling it to bind to DNA or, as shown elsewhere, to nuclei (Kalimi, Beato, and Feigelson, 1973).

If the steroid-receptor complex is kept at 0°C for several hours, its slow conversion to the activated state can be demonstrated as seen in Figure 2. Addition of millimolar levels of

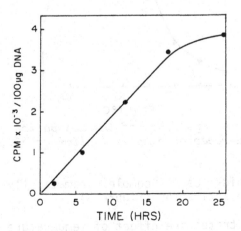

Figure 2.   The slow low temperature activation of steroid-receptor complex (Kalimi et al., 1975).

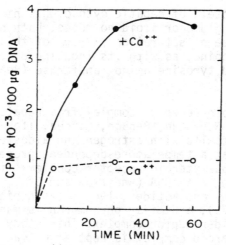

Figure 3.   *Effect of Ca^{++} upon the time course of activation of hormone-receptor complex at low temperature (Kalimi et al., 1975).*

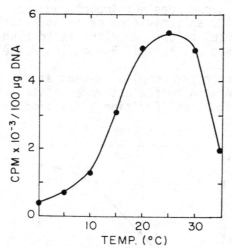

Figure 4.   *Temperature dependence of the activation of the gluco-corticoid-receptor complex (Kalimi et al., 1975).*

calcium to the steroid-receptor complex dramatically accelerates this low-temperature activation (Figure 3).

Figure 4 demonstrates the effect of temperature in the absence of calcium on the activation of the steroid-receptor complex. It is evident that under these *in vitro* conditions, the temperature which

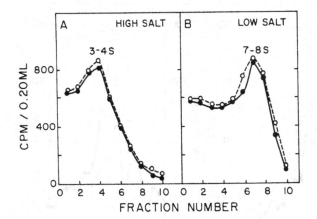

Figure 5. Sucrose density gradient centrifugation of unactivated and thermally activated rat liver cytosol hormone-re- ceptor complexes at low and high ionic strengths. ●---● and O---O represent unactivated and activated cytosol hormone-receptor complexes respectively (Kalimi et al., 1975).

gives the maximum activation is 25°C and that at higher tempera- tures denaturation of the steroid-receptor complex occurs.

The chemical nature of the activation process remains obscure. As seen in Figure 5, the unactivated hormone-receptor complex sedi- ments indistinguishably from the activated complex. At low ionic strength, both complexes sediment as approximately 7-8S species, and at high ionic strength as 3-4S species. For both the activated and unactivated steroid-receptor complexes, increasing the ionic strength brings about a reversible dissociation of the complex to a form with lower sedimentation velocity.

The isoelectric points of the unactivated and activated steroid-receptor complexes were measured. As shown in Figure 6, the unactivated complex has an isoelectric point of 7.1, whereas the thermally activated complex manifests a marked downward shift in its isoelectric point to a pI of 6.1. It remains uncertain whether a temperature-dependent conformational change of the ster- oid-receptor complex is occurring or whether a calcium activatable cytoplasmic enzyme covalently modifies the protein of the steroid- receptor complex. Whatever its precise chemical nature, the trans- formation irreversibly imparts to the steroid-receptor complex the ability to bind to nuclei or to stripped DNA. It is of interest to note that, as shown in Table 4, activation of the steroid-receptor

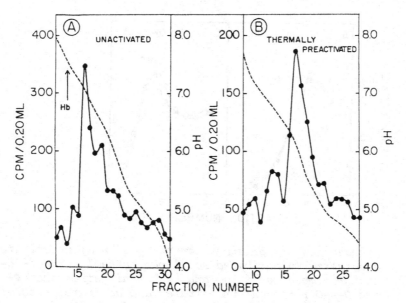

Figure 6. Isoelectric profiles of unactivated and activated [³H] triamcinolone-receptor complexes (Kalimi et al., 1975).

Table 4. BINDING OF UNACTIVATED AND THERMALLY ACTIVATED [³H]-TRI-AMCINOLONE-RECEPTOR COMPLEXES TO CATIONIC AND ANIONIC CELLULOSE MATRICES

Matrix	Nonactivated cytosol	Activated cytosol
	cpm	cpm
DNA-cellulose	390	5282
Phosphocellulose	215	2800
DEAE-cellulose	3884	3163

(Kalimi *et al.*, 1975)

complex also increases its ability to bind to the synthetic negatively charged resin, phosphocellulose, as well as to DNA. Activation does not result, however, in loss of the ability of the complex to bind to positively charged DEAE-cellulose. Thus, the steroid-receptor complex contains regions with negatively charged groups, enabling its binding to DEAE-cellulose, and apparently activation results in the generation of positively charged domains on the steroid-receptor complex, which enable it to bind to DNA, chromatin, nuclei, and phosphocellulose.

A rapid procedure for the purification of the hepatic gluco-corticoid receptor has been developed which exploits the observation that "activation" of this complex enables it to bind to an-ionic substances such as DNA and phosphocellulose (Colman and Feigelson, 1976). The procedure uses two phosphocellulose columns operated in sequence. The first column removes from unfraction-ated cytosol all basic proteins which adhere to the immobilized

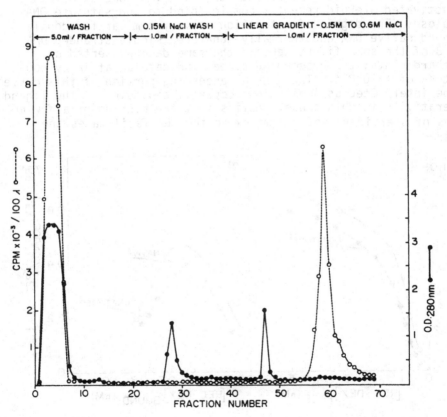

Figure 7. Receptor purification by gradient elution on phospho-cellulose chromatography of the retained thermally activated steroid-receptor complex (Colman and Feigel-son, 1976).

phosphate residues; the unactivated steroid-receptor complex elutes
in the flow-through of this first column. This complex is then
thermally activated and applied to a second phosphocellulose column
where it is retained, washed, and eluted by a salt gradient. As
shown in Figure 7, fractions 56-60 contain purified glucocorticoid-
receptor complex with very low levels of contamination protein.
This simple procedure is capable of purifying the steroid-receptor
complex over 1000-fold.

Quantitative studies have compared the ability of the activated steroid-receptor complex to bind to double stranded (native)
and single stranded (denatured) DNA at low ionic strength. The
degree of saturation of a given amount of DNA affixed to cellulose
was measured as a function of the concentration of activated
steroid-receptor complex. As shown in Figure 8 (Feigelson, Beato,
Colman, Kalimi, Killewich, and Schutz, 1975), nanomolar levels of
the activated steroid-receptor complex bind to and saturate DNA-
cellulose. The degree of saturation is very similar for double
stranded native DNA and thermally denatured single stranded DNA.
Part B of the same figure depicts the same data presented as
Scatchard plots; the descending slopes indicate an affinity constant Ka of $1 \times 10^9 M^{-1}$. The unusual ascending portion of this curve
may be interpreted as indicating cooperative binding of the ligand.
Cooperativity in this sense, implies that the binding of a few molecules of steroid-receptor complex to the DNA facilitates the

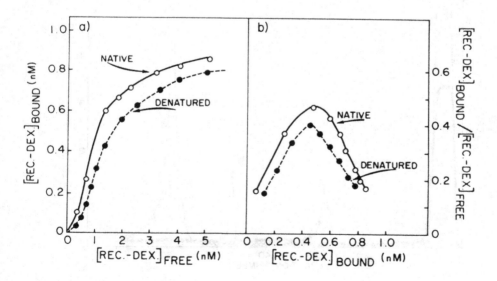

*Figure 8. Binding of activated receptor-dexamethasone complex
(R-D) to native 0---0 and denatured ●---● rat liver
DNA-cellulose (Feigelson et al., 1975).*

binding of further molecules of steroid-receptor complex. Whether this is an artifact of the *in vitro* system, or whether it reflects a fundamental property of the interaction of the steroid-receptor complex with DNA is uncertain.

Metabolic Effects of Glucocorticoids

One of the earliest indications of the biological activity of the glucocorticoids was the stimulation of gluconeogenesis *in vivo* and in liver slices (Koepf, Horn, Gremmill, and Torn, 1941; Long, Katzin, and Frey, 1940). These effects are initiated by the glucocorticoids acting on lymphoid and muscle tissues, resulting in the breakdown of their cellular proteins into amino acids. These amino acids are transported through the blood to the liver, where they undergo transamination and deamination. The amino groups are converted to urea and excreted. The carbon skeletons of the glucogenic amino acids enter carbohydrate metabolism and are converted by gluconeogenesis to hepatic glycogen or blood glucose. In addition, these hormones act directly on hepatocytes, stimulating gluconeogenesis (Haynes, 1965; Long *et al.*, 1940) and induce elevated levels of certain enzymes involved in amino acid metabolism, e.g., tryptophan oxygenase and tyrosine transaminase (Baxter and Tomkins, 1970; Feigelson, Feigelson, and Greengard, 1962; Goldstein, Stella, and Knox, 1962; Kenney and Flora, 1961). Immunochemical titrations indicate that hormonal increases of hepatic enzyme activity were accompanied by increased enzyme protein levels (Feigelson and Greengard, 1962; Kenney, 1962). This was followed by the demonstration that the hormone increases the rate of labeled amino acid incorporation into the inducible enzymes *in vivo* (Schimke, Sweeney, and Berlin, 1965) and *in vitro* (Granner, Hayashi, Thompson, and Tomkins, 1968). In addition, the treatment of animals (Greengard and Acs, 1962) or hepatoma cells (Peterkofsky and Tomkins, 1967) with Actinomycin D, puromycin, or cycloheximide prevented enzyme induction by the steroids, demonstrating that the steroids, in a transcriptionally dependent process, selectively increase the rate of synthesis of certain hepatic enzymes.

Control of Specific Species of mRNA by Glucocorticoids

The participation of RNA in several capacities during protein synthesis prompted studies into the effects of glucocorticoids on the biosynthesis of RNA during the course of hormonal induction of hepatic enzymes. It was shown that the incorporation of radioactive precursor into liver RNA is markedly stimulated following cortisol administration (Feigelson, Feigelson, and Greengard, 1960; Feigelson, Gross, and Feigelson, 1962). The time course of this stimulation in RNA metabolism parallels that of the induction of tryptophan oxygenase by the hormone (Feigelson and Feigelson, 1965). Further studies indicated hormonally increased rates of synthesis of both ribosomal and mRNA *in vivo* (Hanoune and Feigelson, 1969; Yu and Feigelson, 1969).

Selected regions of the genome are transcribed by RNA polymerase II into the nuclear precursors of the various messenger RNAs.
The heterogeneous nuclear RNAs are processed by hydrolytic cleavage,
base modification, and adenylation. They are then transported to
the cytoplasm where as mRNA they act as templates for protein synthesis. Until recently it was not known at what stage the glucocorticoid hormones act in this complex series of events. Sex
steroidal effects upon rates of transcription and stabilization of
the messenger RNA have been proposed (Chan, Means, and O'Malley,
1973; Palmiter and Carey, 1974). It has been considered that glucocorticoids may be implicated in the action of a cytoplasmic re-
pressor of messenger RNA (Tomkins, Gelehrter, Granner, Martin,
Samuels, and Thompson, 1969). To distinguish between these various hypotheses, we measured the level of messenger RNA for one
hormonally-inducible protein, tryptophan oxygenase, to determine
whether the increased rate of synthesis of this enzyme protein following hormonal administration was due to a rise in the tissue
levels of its functional messenger RNA or to a hormonally-mediated
increased translational efficiency of a fixed level of this messenger RNA. To answer this question, it was necessary to develop
an assay for the messenger RNA for tryptophan oxygenase. The messenger RNA was first partially purified by binding its polyA sequences to cellulose columns (Kitos, Saxon, and Amos, 1972; Schutz
et al., 1972) enabling its separation from the other species of
cellular RNA (Figure 9). At hgih ionic strength, ribosomal RNA and
transfer RNA do not bind to cellulose. Lowering the ionic strength
elutes about 2% of the total RNA, which was shown by polyU hybridization and translocational activity to consist of polyA-containing
messenger RNA (Sipple, Stavrianopoulos, Schutz and Feigelson, 1974).
Microgram levels of messenger RNA prepared in this manner from rat
liver, when added to a modified cellfree Krebs II ascites system
(Mathews and Rosner, 1970) stimulated the incorporation of tritiated leucine into tryptophan oxygenase. The mRNA preparations
were incubated for one hour in the fortified Krebs ribosomal system. After the incubation, the ribosomes were removed by centrifugation, and the supernatant containing the newly synthesized
radioactive polypeptides was collected. Tryptophan oxygenase was
isolated from the released chains by immunoprecipitation with carrier tryptophan oxygenase and monospecific antitryptophan oxygenase, followed by SDS-polyacrylamide gel electrophoresis of the
solubilized immunoprecipitate. The gels were stained for protein,
enabling identification of the various protein markers which had
been added, sliced, and the radioactivity determined by liquid
scintillation techniques. A radioactive peak was observed, as
shown in Figure 10, at the gel position corresponding to 43,000
Daltons, which is the molecular weight of both subunits of tryptophan oxygenase. Thus, the radioactivity which appears on the gel
at this position is coded for by hepatic mRNA, is immunoprecip-

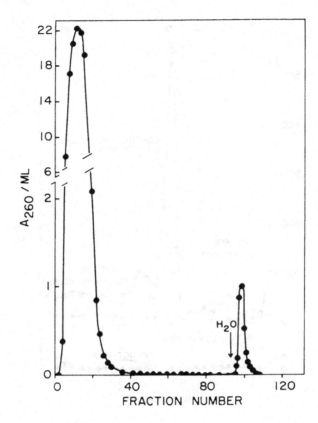

*Figure 9. Chromatography on cellulose of polysomal RNA (Schutz
et al., 1972).*

itated by specific antibodies to tryptophan oxygenase, and has a
molecular weight which corresponds to the molecular weight of the
protomeric units of hepatic tryptophan oxygenase (Schutz *et al.*,
1973). We, therefore, infer that we are indeed observing a messenger RNA-dependent synthesis of tryptophan oxygenase.

It is known that after the administration of an inducing dose
of steroid, synthesis of the inducible enzymes is enhanced for a
few hours and then returns to control levels. Estimation of the
level of functional mRNA for tryptophan oxygenase in livers of
animals during the induction and deinduction phases indicates that
during the period of increasing enzyme synthesis the level of the
mRNA for tryptophan oxygenase is proportionately increased. During
deinduction, when the enzyme level falls, the mRNA level is also

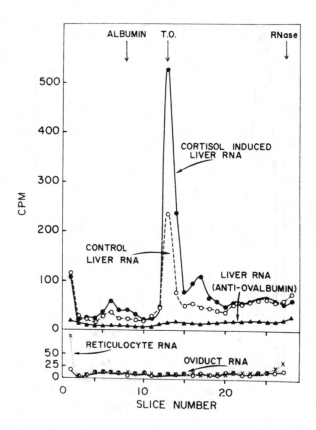

Figure 10.   *The mRNA dependent translational synthesis of trypto-*
phan oxygenase. Upper panel: proteins directed by
liver mRNA from uninduced animals 0---0, and by liver
mRNA from animals that had received hydrocortisone
●---● were precipitated with carrier tryptophan oxygen-
ase and anti-tryptophan oxygenase. Another sample
stimulated by liver mRNA from induced animals was pre-
cipitated with chicken ovalbumin and anti-ovalbumin
▲---▲. Lower panel: proteins directed by cellulose-
purified mRNA from rabbit reticulocytes X---X and RNA
from chicken oviducts 0---0 were precipitated with car-
rier tryptophan oxygenase and anti-tryptophan oxygenase.
Arrows indicate the position of proteins used as in-
ternal markers in the sodium dodecyle sulfate-acryla-
mide gel electrophoresis (Schutz, et al., 1973).

found to decrease (Figures 11 and 12). To confirm and extend
these studies, the level of the mRNA for tryptophan oxygenase and
relative enzyme activities were compared at a fixed induction time

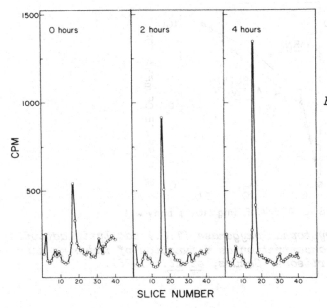

Figure 11. Sodium do-
  decyl sulfate-poly-
  acrylamide electro-
  phoresis of trypto-
  phan oxygenase syn-
  thesized *in vitro*
  (Schutz, Killewich,
  Chen, and Feigelson,
  1975).

Figure 12. Comparison of
  tryptophan osygenase
  catalytic activity with
  mRNA levels for trypto-
  phan oxygenase in the
  livers of rats as a
  function of time after
  intraperitoneal admin-
  istration of hydrocor-
  tisone (Schutz *et al.*
  1975).

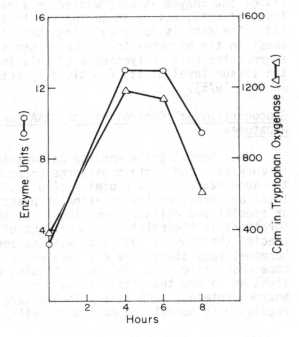

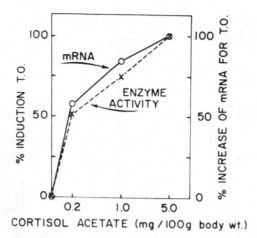

Figure 13. *Hepatic tryptophan oxygenase (T.O.) catalytic activity*
and mRNA concentration as a function of inducing dose
of hydrocortisone (Schutz, et al., 1975).

following administration of increasing doses of steroid. The
rise in enzyme activity, reflecting an increased rate of synthesis of the enzyme is accompanied by a parallel increase in the
level of mRNA, active in coding for tryptophan oxygenase (Figure
13). The data is now convincing that glucocorticoid hormones, at
least in the hormonal induction of hepatic tryptophan oxygenase,
augment the rate of synthesis of this inducible enzyme by elevating
the tissue level of its functionally active messenger RNA (Schutz
et al., 1975).

Glucocorticoidal Control of the mRNA for Tryptophan Oxygenase in Hepatomas

When normal cells undergo malignant transformation alterations,
in enzymatic and protein patterns occur. These alterations may be
the appearance of new proteins (Abelev, 1971), e.g., the carcino-
fetal antigens, or the deletion of preexistent proteins, enzymes,
or specialized cellular functions. Furthermore, quantitative alterations in the relative proportions of enzymes and isoenzymic
species (Weinhouse, 1972), as well as aberrant responsiveness to
hormonal regulators have all been reported when normal tissues become neoplastic. The following studies were conducted to gain insight as to how the genes coding for the synthesis of specific
enzyme proteins, such as tryptophan oxygenase, are expressed and
regulated in normal and malignant cells.

We prepared total messenger RNA from host livers and hepatomas

Table 5. THE LEVELS OF THE CATALYTIC ACTIVITY AND THE MESSENGER RNA FOR TRYPTOPHAN OXYGENASE IN HOST LIVER AND HEPATOMA

Tissue	Treatment	Tryptophan oxygenase catalytic activity (μmol of kynurenine/hr/gm of liver)	Heterogeneous assay of mRNA-(A)$_x$ (counts per minutes incorporated)			
			Total protein (cpm x 10^6)	Total released chains (cpm x 10^6)	Tryptophan oxygenase (cpm)	% of total protein synthesis
Host liver 7793	none	3.1	5.39	1.35	337	0.025
Host liver 7793	hydrocort.	10.6	5.85	1.89	931	0.069
Hepatoma 7793	none	undetectable	5.42	1.90	undetectable	--
Hepatoma 7793	hydrocort.	undetectable	5.89	1.35	undetectable	--
Host liver 5123C	none	4.9	4.74	1.31	253	0.019
Host liver 5123C	hydrocort.	15.8	5.51	1.45	504	0.034
Hepatoma 5123C	none	undetectable	3.86	1.24	undetectable	--
Hepatoma 5123C	hydrocort.	undetectable	4.41	1.34	undetectable	--
Host liver 5123D	none	4.5	3.81	1.25	261	0.020
Host liver 5123D	hydrocort.	18.0	4.36	1.36	453	0.032
Hepatoma 5123D	none	undetectable	5.29	1.71	undetectable	--
Hepatoma 5123D	hydrocort.	undetectable	6.14	1.91	undetectable	--

(Ramanarayanan-Murthy, Colman, and Feigelson, 1976)

of animals bearing Morris Hepatoma tumors and from host livers
and hepatomas of Morris hepatoma-bearing animals that had received an inducing dose of cortisol four hours prior to sacrifice. As shown in Table 5, 60 µg of poly (A) containing hepatic
messenger RNA from the control tumor-bearing animals led, in 60
minutes, to the incorporation of more than five million cpm of
tritiated leucine into the total protein synthesized in this
translational system. Approximately 25% of this total incorporation existed as released chains, of which 337 cpm of ^{3}H-leucine
were incorporated into tryptophan oxygenase subunits. An identical amount of hepatic mRNA derived from hepatoma-bearing animals which received hydrocortisone four hours prior to sacrifice,
coded for three times as much incorporation into nascent tryptophan oxygenase. In contrast, the mRNA isolated from the hepatomas of control and hormone-treated animals did not show any
incorporation into tryptophan oxygenase subunits indicating the
absence of detectable levels of this mRNA species in the hepatomas of control and hormone-treated animals. It is of interest to note that the hepatic mRNA and hepatoma mRNA of control
and hormone-treated animals do not cause detectably different
rates of amino acid incorporation into the total protein, nor
into the total released chains. It is only after one has suc-
ceeded in separating the protomeric units of tryptophan oxygenase from the total hepatic protein synthesized that one can detect the hormonal elevation in tryptophan oxygenase. Hepatoma
mRNA from either control or hormone-treated animals did not
code for amino acid incorporation into tryptophan oxygenase. On
the basis of this functional assay for messenger RNA we infer
that the level of functional mRNA for tryptophan oxygenase is
about 0.03% and 0.10% of the total hepatic mRNA activity in control and hormone-treated animals respectively (Figure 14). The
level of functional mRNA for tryptophan oxygenase in hepatoma
is undetectably low in control and hormone treated animals. The
absence of this mRNA species could ensue from several causes:
(a) the genes for tryptophan oxygenase in hepatoma may have been
cytogenetically deleted during the malignant transformation, (b)
the genes for tryptophan oxygenase in hepatoma may be transcriptionally silent and not being expressed, or (c) there may be impaired processing of the gene transcript to functionally active
mRNA. Experiments to distinguish between these alternatives are
underway.

The lack of tryptophan oxygenase in hepatoma and its fail-
ure to be induced by glucocorticoids, prompted investigations
on the qualitative and quantitative nature of the functional glucocorticoid receptor in the hepatomas. Our studies indicate that
hepatoma cytosol contains approximately 200 fmoles of receptor
per mg protein, a specific activity which is comparable with its
host liver (Table 6). Also, incubation of purified nuclei with
hepatoma cytosol receptor yielded no significant difference in

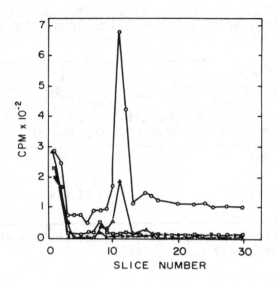

Figure 14. *Evaluation of the synthesis* in vitro *of tryptophan*
oxygenase protomers by mRNA derived *from host livers*
and 7793 Morris hepatomas. ▲---▲ *from control host*
liver mRNA; □---□ *from control tumor RNA; X---X from*
hydrocortisone induced host-liver mRNA; 0---0 from
hydrocortisone induced tumor mRNA (Ramanarayanan-
Murthy et al.*, 1976).*

Table 6. *GLUCOCORTICOID RECEPTOR ACTIVITY IN LIVER AND MORRIS*
HEPATOMA CYTOSOLS

Source of cytosol	Specific bound [^{3}H]-triamcinolone (cpm/mg protein)	% Nonspecific binding
Host liver	2286	25
Morris hepatoma 7793	2339	17

(Ramanarayanan-Murthy *et al.*, 1976)

nuclear uptake when compared with its host liver cytosol (Table
7); in addition, hepatoma derived steroid-receptor complex bound
to stripped rat liver DNA as well as host liver steroid-receptor
complex did (Table 8). Thus the inability of these hepatomas to
respond to glucocorticoids does not seem to be due to the absence

Table 7.   THE BINDING OF LIVER AND MORRIS HEPATOMA CYTOPLASMIC GLU-
COCORTICOID RECEPTOR COMPLEXES TO HOMOLOGOUS AND HETERO-
LOGOUS NUCLEI

Source of nuclei	[³H]TA-host liver receptor complex		[³H]TA-hepatoma receptor complex	
	Specific bound [³H]TA (cpm/mg DNA)	% Nonspecif- ic binding	Specific bound [³H]TA (cpm/mg DNA)	% Nonspecif- ic binding
Host liver	57,371	38	77,214	22
Morris hepatoma 7793	67,143	18	72,814	18

[³H]TA=Triamcinolone acetonide (Sp. Act. 16 Ci/mmole)
(Ramanarayanan-Murthy *et al.*, 1976)

Table 8.   THE BINDING OF LIVER AND MORRIS HEPATOMA CYTOPLASMIC GLU-
COCORTICOID RECEPTOR COMPLEXES TO RAT LIVER DNA-CELLULOSE

Source of cytosol	Specific bound [³H]TA (cpm/100 μg DNA)	% Nonspecific binding
Host liver	7090	7.8
Morris hepatoma 7793	6966	9.7

[³H]TA=Triamcinolone acetonide (Sp. Act. 16 Ci/mmole)
(Ramanarayanan-Murthy *et al.*, 1976)

of the glucocorticoid receptor or to any detectable impaired functional interaction with nuclei (Ramanarayanan-Murthy *et al.*, 1976).

Interaction of the Receptor with Nuclear Components

The pioneering studies of Mueller and his colleagues on estrogen action on RNA and protein synthesis very early linked hormone
action with gene expression (Mueller, Herranen, and Jervell, 1958).
The microbial analogy of a repressor-gene interaction was quickly
absorbed into the concept of steroid hormone action. This had led
to a search for the specific components or acceptors that bind the
hormone receptor complex in the nucleus. Our recent studies demonstrate that treatment of rat liver nuclei with DNase-I or staphylo-
coccal nuclease causing them to lose even 10% of the nuclear DNA,

results in a loss of about 80% of their capacity to bind glucocorticoid receptor complex at low ionic strength. Thus, the steroid-receptor complex binds to a small portion of the genome which is readily sensitive to DNase (manuscript in preparation).

Conclusions

It has been experimentally demonstrated that the glucocorticoid hormone, after entering the cell, interacts with a receptor protein in the cytosol to form a glucocorticoid-receptor complex. This complex undergoes activation of unknown molecular nature, rendering it capable of entry into the nucleus where it interacts with specific sites on the genome. It is also known that a rise in the tissue level of functionally active specific mRNA for tryptophan oxygenase accompanies and seems to be responsible for the hormonally-induced increased rate of synthesis of this enzyme (Feigelson *et al.*, 1975). What can not be definitively excluded at the present time are glucocorticoidal effects upon mRNA levels which may be mediated through selective alterations in processing or transport of specific mRNA species. However, the most likely interpretation of the data on hand, is that steroid hormones mediate a steroid-receptor-genomic interaction which accelerates transcription of a relatively small number of specific genes. Each structural gene, which codes for a specific protein, represents less than one part in a million of the total base-pairs in the mammalian genome. The majority of the 10^4 cellular receptor molecules found in the nucleus may be bound non-specifically to the genome. A fundamental question, which remains to be answered, is how the great selectivity in receptor action is achieved in spite of an apparently weak selectivity in receptor binding to nuclei. Our recent studies indicate the existence of two types of receptor binding sites on the genome. The DNase sensitive binding sites and the DNase-resistant binding sites. The physiological importance of these two types of binding sites is under current investigation.

REFERENCES

Abelev, G.I. (1971) Alpha-fetoprotein in ontogenesis and its association with malignant tumors. *Adv. in Cancer Res.*, 14:295-358.

Anderson, K.M. and Liao, S. (1968) Selective retention of dihydrotestosterone by prostatic nuclei. *Nature*, 219:277-279.

Baxter, J.D. and Tomkins, G.M. (1970) The relationship between glucocorticoid binding and tyrosine aminotransferase induction in hepatoma tissue culture cells. *Proc. Nat'l. Acad. Sci. USA*, 65: 709-715.

Baxter, J.D., Rousseau, G.G., Benson, M.C., Garcea, R.L., Ito, J. and Tomkins, G.M. (1972) Role of DNA and specific cytoplasmic receptors in glucocorticoid action. *Proc. Nat'l. Acad. Sci. USA*, 69:1892-1896.

Beato, M. and Feigelson, P. (1972) Glucocorticoid-binding proteins
    of rat liver cytosol. 1. Separation and identification of
    the binding proteins. *J. Biol. Chem.*, 247:7890-7896.

Beato, M., Kalimi, M., and Feigelson, P. (1972) Correlation be-
    tween glucocorticoid binding to specific liver cytosol re-
    ceptors and enzyme induction *in vivo*. *Biochem. Biophys. Res.
    Commun.*, 47:1464-1472.

Beato, M., Kalimi, M., Beato, W., and Feigelson, P. (1974) Inter-
    action of glucocorticoids with rat liver nuclei: Effect of
    adrenalectomy and cortisol administration. *Endocrinology*,
    94:377-387.

Chan, L., Means, A.R., and O'Malley, B.W. (1973) Rates of induc-
    tion of specific translatable messenger RNAs for ovalbumin
    and avidin by steroid hormones. *Proc. Nat'l. Acad. Sci. USA*,
    70:1870-1874.

Colman, P.D. and Feigelson, P. (1976) Purification of the acti-
    vated glucocorticoid-receptor complex. *Mol. Cell Endocrinol.*,
    5:33-40.

Feigelson, M. and Feigelson, P. (1965) Metabolic effects of gluco-
    corticoids as related to enzyme induction. *Advances Enzy.
    Regul.*, 3:11-27.

Feigelson, M., Gross, P., and Feigelson, P. (1962) Early effects
    of cortisone on nucleic acid and protein metabolism of rat
    liver. *Biochim. Biophys. Acta*, 55:495-504.

Feigelson, P., Beato, M., Colman, P., Kalimi, M., Killewich, L.A.,
    and Schutz, G. (1975) Studies on the hepatic glucocorticoid
    receptor and on the hormonal modulation of specific mRNA
    levels during enzyme induction. *Rec. Prog. Horm. Res.*, 31:
    213-242.

Feigelson, P., Feigelson, M., and Greengard, O. (1962) Comparison
    of the mechanisms of hormonal and substrate induction of rat
    liver tryptophan pyrrolase. *Rec. Prog. Horm. Res.*, 18:491-512.

Feigelson, P. and Greengard, O. (1962) Immunochemical evidence for
    increased titers of liver tryptophan pyrrolase during substrate
    and hormonal enzyme induction. *J. Biol. Chem.*, 237:3714-3717.

Feldman, D., Funder, J.W., and Edelman, I.S. (1972) Subcellular
    mechanisms in the action of adrenal steroids. *Amer. J. Med.*,
    53:545-560.

Goldstein, L., Stella, E.J., and Knox, W.E. (1962) The effect of
    hydrocortisone on tyrosine-α-ketoglutarate transaminase and
    tryptophan pyrrolase activities in the isolated, perfused rat
    liver. *J. Biol. Chem.*, 237:1723-1726.

Gorski, J., Toft, D., Shyamala, G., Smith, D., and Notides, A.
    (1968) Hormone receptors: Studies on the interaction of
    estrogen with the uterus. *Rec. Prog. Horm. Res.*, 24:45-80.

Granner, D.K., Hayashi, S., Thompson, E.B., and Tomkins, G.M.
    (1968) Stimulation of tyrosine aminotransferase synthesis by
    dexamethasone phosphate in cell culture. *J. Mol. Biol.*, 35:
    291-301.

Greengard, O. and Acs, G. (1962) The effect of actinomycin on the substrate and hormonal induction of liver enzymes. *Biochim. Biophys. Acta*, 61:652-653.

Hanoune, J. and Feigelson, P. (1969) Turnover of protein and RNA of liver ribosomal components in normal and cortisol-treated rats. *Biochim. Biophys. Acta*, 199:214-223.

Haynes, R.C. Jr. (1965) The control of gluconeogenesis by adrenal cortical hormones. *Advan. in Enzyme Regul.*, 3:111-119.

Jensen, E.V. and DeSombre, E.R. (1973) Estrogen-receptor interaction: Estrogenic hormones effect transformation of specific receptor proteins to a biochemically functional form. *Science*, 182:127-134.

Jensen, E.V. and Jacobson, H.I. (1962) Basic guides to the mechanism of estrogen action. *Rec. Prog. Horm. Res.*, 18:387-414.

Kalimi, M., Colman, P., and Feigelson, P. (1975) The "activated" hepatic glucocorticoid-receptor complex: Its generation and properties. *J. Biol. Chem.*, 250:1080-1086.

Kalimi, M. Beato, M., and Feigelson, P. (1973) Interaction of glucocorticoids with rat liver nuclei. 1. Role of the cytosol proteins. *Biochemistry*, 12:3365-3371.

Kenney, F.T. (1962) Induction of tyrosine-α-ketoglutarate transaminase in rat liver. IV. Evidence for an increase in the rate of enzyme synthesis. *J. Biol. Chem.*, 236:3495-3498.

Kenney, F.T. and Flora, R.M. (1961) Induction of tyrosine-α-ketoglutarate transaminase in rat liver. I. Hormonal nature. *J. Biol. Chem.*, 236:2699-2702.

King, R.J.B. and Mainwaring, W.I.P. (1974) *Steroid-cell interactions*. Baltimore: University Park Press.

Kitos, P.A., Saxon, G., and Amos, H. (1972) The isolation of polyadenylate with unreacted cellulose. *Biochim. Biophys. Res. Commun.*, 46:1426-1437.

Koblinsky, M. (1973) Doctoral Dissertation. Columbia University, New York.

Koblinsky, M., Beato, M., Kalimi, M., and Feigelson, P. (1972) Glucocorticoid-binding proteins of rat liver cytosol. II. Physical characterization and properties of the binding proteins. *J. Biol. Chem.*, 247:7897-7904.

Koepf, G.F., Horn, H.W., Gemmill, C.L., and Thorn, G.W. (1941) The effect of adrenal cortical hormone on the synthesis of carbohydrate in liver slices. *Amer. J. Physiol.*, 135:175-186.

Long, C.N.H., Katzin, B., and Frey, E.G. (1940) The adrenal cortex and carbohydrate metabolism. *Endocrinology*, 26:309-344.

Mathews, M.B. and Korner, A. (1970) Mammalian cell-free protein synthesis directed by viral ribonucleic acid. *Eur. J. Biochem.*, 17:328-338.

Mueller, G.C., Herranen, A.M., and Jervell, K.F. (1958) Studies on the mechanism of action of estrogens. *Rec. Prog. Horm. Res.*, 14:95-139.

O'Malley, B.W. and Means, A.R. (1974) Female steroid hormones and target cell nuclei. *Science*, 183:610-620.

Palmiter, R.D. and Carey, N.H. (1974) Rapid inactivation of oval-
    bumin messenger ribonucleic acid after acute withdrawal of
    estrogen. *Proc. Nat'l. Acad. Sci. USA*, 71:2357-2361.
Peterkofsky, B. and Tomkins, G.M. (1967) Effect of inhibitors of
    nucleic acid synthesis on steroid-mediated induction of tyro-
    sine aminotransferase in hepatoma cell cultures. *J. Mol.
    Biol.*, 30:49-61.
Ramanarayanan-Murthy, L. Colman, P.D., Morris, H.P., and Feigelson,
    P. (1976) Pretranslational control of tryptophan oxygenase
    levels in Morris hepatoma and host liver. *Cancer Res.*, 36:
    3594-3599.
Schimke, R.T., Sweeney, E.W., and Berlin, C.M. (1964) An analysis
    of the kinetics of rat liver tryptophan pyrrolase induction:
    The significance of both enzyme synthesis and degradation.
    Biochem. Biophys. Res. Commun., 15:214-219.
Schutz, G., Beato, M., and Feigelson, P. (1973) Messenger RNA for
    hepatic tryptophan oxygenase: Its partial purification, its
    translation in a heterologous cell-free system, and its con-
    trol by glucocorticoid hormones. *Proc. Nat'l. Acad. Sci. USA*,
    70:1218-1221.
Schutz, G., Beato, M., and Feigelson, P. (1972) Isolation of eu-
    karyotic messenger RNA on cellulose and its translocation *in
    vitro*. *Biochem. Biophys. Res. Commun.*, 49:680-689.
Schutz, G., Killewich, L., Chen, G., and Feigelson, P. (1975) Con-
    trol of the mRNA for hepatic tryptophan oxygenase during hor-
    monal and substrate induction. *Proc. Nat'l. Acad. Sci. USA*,
    72:1017-1020.
Sippel, A.E., Stavrianopoulos, J.G., Schutz, G., and Feigelson, P.
    (1974) Translational properties of rabbit globin mRNA after
    specific removal of poly(A) with ribonuclease H. *Proc. Nat'l.
    Acad. Sci. USA*, 71:4635-4639.
Tomkins, G.M., Gelehrter, T.D., Granner, D, Martin, D. Jr., Samuels,
    H.H., and Thompson, E.B. (1969) Control of specific gene ex-
    pression in higher organisms. Expression of mammalian genes
    may be controlled by repressors acting on the translation of
    messenger RNA. *Science*, 166:1474-1480.
Weinhouse, S. (1972) Glycolysis, respiration, and anomalous gene
    expression in experimental hepatomas: G.H.A. Clowes Memorial
    Lecture. *Cancer Res.*, 32:2007-2016.
Westphal, U. (1971) *Steroid-protein interactions*. New York:
    Springer-Verlag, Monographs on Endocrinology, Vol. 4.
Yu, F-L and Feigelson, P. (1969) The sequential stimulation of
    uracil-rich and guanine-rich RNA species during cortisone in-
    duction of hepatic enzymes. *Biochem. Biophys. Res. Commun.*,
    35:499-504.

ACKNOWLEDGMENT

These studies were supported in part by grants CA 02332 and CRTY 05011 from the National Cancer Institute of the National Institutes of Health.

DEDICATION

One of us (LRM) wishes to dedicate this review to the fond memory of her beloved father, Shri Gundlupet Sadashiv Dakshinamurthy, who expired during the preparation of this manuscript, for his inspiration and encouragement to attain the highest standards in scholarship.

DISCUSSION AFTER DR. FEIGELSON'S TALK

Dr. Hechter
    This is an elegant contribution to the action of glucocorti-
coids in liver, which has significantly clarified this field. Have
you been able to isolate and directly measure the messenger RNA
for tryptophan oxygenase, whose synthesis is increased by the glucocorticoid-receptor complex?

Dr. Feigelson
    Not yet. We are presently struggling to develop procedures
which will enable us to purify trace mRNA species such as that for
tryptophan oxygenase. Should we succeed then it will be easy to
prepare a cDNA employing viral reverse transcriptase. With a specific cDNA probe in hand it will then become possible to explore
the important questions you have raised. [Added in proof: We
have recently developed procedures for purification of trace mRNA
species and preparation of the corresponding pure cDNA: D. Kurtz
and P. Feigelson in *Nucleic Acid Research*, 4:71-84 (1977).]

Dr. Franz
    Is it true that with your present technology you cannot dis-
tinguish between an activation of preformed messenger RNA for
tryptophan oxygenase versus the *de novo* synthesis of additional
messenger RNA for tryptophan oxygenase?

Dr. Feigelson
    That is correct. We are in the same position as someone who
observes an increase in enzymatic activity but who has no specific
antibody to measure the amount of enzyme protein. An increase in
enzymic activity could reflect increased number of enzyme molecules
or conversion to a more active form. In the absence of a specific
cDNA to enable quantitation of the base sequences for a specific
mRNA we cannot definitely distinguish between activation or increase in this mRNA species. It is worth remembering that hormonal
enzyme induction is prevented by α-amanitin which inhibits gene
transcription. It is, therefore, probable that hormonal enzyme
induction is via hormonal enhancement of specific gene transcription leading to a rise in the level of the corresponding mRNA and
a consequent increased synthesis of the induced enzyme.

Dr. Kornel
    It's very elegant and impressive work, Dr. Feigelson. I have
a few other technical questions in chronological order of your
presentation. You discussed the enhancement of the uptake of dexamethasone into isolated nuclei by the addition of cytosol or specific receptor protein. You also mentioned that the addition of
transcortin did not increase the nuclear uptake of dexamethasone.
However, transcortin doesn't bind dexamethasone.

Dr. Feigelson
    We've done similar experiments with labeled corticosterone
and cortisol. Neither transcortin nor cytosol fractions free of
glucocorticoid receptor will translocate these steroids to nuclei
in vitro, whereas fractions of cytosol that contain the glucocorticoid receptor will not only bind steroids but also evoke nuclear
binding.

Dr. Kornel
    Then the next question. I know it is generally accepted that
there is a translocation of the receptor-steroid complex to the
nucleus from cytoplasm.

Dr. Feigelson
    Don't generally accept anything in this field.

Dr. Kornel
    It is assumed, though. My question is whether anybody, in-
cluding yourself, actually experimented with labeled receptor,
not only via tritium labelling of the steroid moiety, but labelling the receptor protein itself with iodine or another radio-
isotope.

Dr. Feigelson
    As we do not have absolutely homogeneous glucocorticoid re-
ceptor we cannot perform that direct experiment.

Dr. Kornel
    So there is really no absolute evidence that there is true,
translocation of the receptor?

Dr. Feigelson
    There is no <u>absolute</u> evidence for this subcellular transloca-
tion of receptor <u>but there</u> is reasonably convincing evidence that
it does take place. This includes our study with cytosol prepared
from adrenalectomized animals incubated with and without glucocorticoid and then exposed to nuclei. Following removal of nuclei by
centrifugation, assaying the concentration of residual cytoplasmic
glucocorticoid receptor indicates that this decreases only when
steroid had been added to the incubation mixture. Thus, receptor
translocates to nuclei only when it exists as steroid-receptor
complex.

Dr. Kornel
    In your studies of the binding to deoxyribonuclease-treated
nuclei, you have shown that there remains some residual binding of
the activated steroid receptor complex. Do you conclude that this
binding is to nuclear protein?

Dr. Feigelson
    Yes, to residual nucleo-protein.

Dr. Kornel
    If so, is it an acidic protein rather than histone? This is
the general consensus I believe.

Dr. Feigelson
    It's binding to the nucleo-protein complex; I'm not indi-
cating it's binding just to the protein. It's binding to what's
left after partial DNAse hydrolysis. These are clipped nucleo-
somes which contain nuclear proteins and DNA. I have not dissect-
ed any further.

Dr. Kornel
    There are in the liver, of course, many glucocorticoid-bind-
ing proteins.

Dr. Feigelson
    We have detected only one dexamethasone-binding protein.

Dr. Kornel
    There is intracellular transcortin in the liver.

Dr. Feigelson
    It doesn't bind dexamethasone.

Dr. Kornel
    Yes, I didn't specifically mention dexamethasone but gluco-
corticoid-binding proteins. I recall your earlier work and it was
then confirmed by our work. We used affinity chromatography to
isolate glucocorticoid-binding proteins from the liver (Wong, Kornel, Bezkorovainy, and Murphy, 1973) and we could show that there
are at least three different proteins in the liver that bind cortisol or corticosterone. Subsequent to the binding and the incubation of the protein-steroid preparation, you could extract from
that protein intact steroid, proving that these are not proteins
involved in the metabolism of the steroid (enzymes). This was
shown also by Beato, who used different techniques for the isolation of these proteins from rat liver, and who, I believe, was
working with you. Now, I would appreciate it if you could comment
on this--what do you think may be the role of these one or two proteins that bind corticoids but still do not cause any transformation of the molecular structure of that particular steroid?

Dr. Feigelson
    We detect three glucocorticoid-binding proteins. One of
these also binds dexamethasone and is, for the reasons I've given
earlier, believed to be the functional glucocorticoid receptor.
The second protein found in the hepatic cytosol is transcortin,

which is synthesized in the liver and secreted into the plasma.
Its function is believed to be as an extracellular glucocorticoid
transport protein. The third glucocorticoid-binding protein also
does not bind dexamethasone, does bind natural glucocorticoids
and cross reacts with antibodies prepared against serum transcortin. We have no idea concerning its functional role.

Dr. Kornel
     There has been one postulate, by Beato and Sekeris, I be-
lieve, that these two other proteins, from which intact cortisol
can be extracted following the binding, serve as the steroid-de-
pot. In other words, they prevent a certain amount of the steroid
in the liver from being metabolized by the enzymes which are also
present in the same cells. Do you think this is tenable?

Dr. Feigelson
     I don't know the answer to that.

Dr. Hechter
     I don't know that you can answer the following question, but
I'm sure you've thought about it. Let us assume that the steroid-
receptor complex once activated (perhaps by a divalent cation),
"goes" to acceptor sites in the nucleus; in consequence, specific
mRNA's are synthesized and released into the cytoplasm. With glucocorticoids, this process occurs in the thymus, as well as the
liver and a variety of other tissues. In each case, a set of proteins are synthesized which are appropriate to the glucocorticoid
message received. The question then arises: how do you control
this process so that a single moiety--the steroid-receptor complex
--goes to the "right" regions on the genome to "read-out" a new
set of genes which differ depending on the cell types involved?
In effect, a single mechanism is postulated to achieve expression
of different gene sets. I would appreciate it if you would share
with us your thinking about this aspect of steroid hormone action.

Dr. Feigelson
     Oscar, you've put your finger on the key question for all of
us for the next ten years. You've formulated the problem of differentiation. One possibility is that each cell contains many
different *sigma* factors so that RNA polymerase II is directed to
specific genes. I consider this less likely than there being tissue-specific proteins on the genome, which select and determine
the genomic sites, to which steroid-receptor complexes bind and
at which RNA polymerase II can initiate transcription.

Dr. Lefkowitz
     You mentioned early in your talk that the specificity, in
terms of the ability of various steroids to compete for these
dexamethasone sites, was very similar to what one would like, but
there were a few discrepancies that bothered you, and then you

didn't go into them. As I recall, you mentioned that there were
some compounds which would inhibit this binding but which didn't
appear to have the physiological effects you'd expect them to
have. Do you know whether those compounds would, in fact, be
antagonists of the physiological effects of dexamethasone?

Dr. Feigelson
    Oscar Hechter would know this better than I do. Progesterone
is a reasonably good competing agent, yet, I believe it does not
have good glucocorticoid activity.

Dr. Lefkowitz
    But do you know whether they would competitively inhibit the
glucocorticoids?

Dr. Feigelson
    I don't know the physiological effectiveness of progesterone
as a glucocorticoid antagonist.

Dr. Heimberg
    I guess one of the questions that we all are struggling with
is to find out when you're going to have a purified *in vitro* system where you can make your messenger RNA.

Dr. Feigelson
    You're going to hear that from our next speaker.

Dr. Heimberg
    Are you going to talk about that too?

Dr. Feigelson
    Sure. In a few years.

DISCUSSION REFERENCES

Wong, K.C., Kornel, L., Bezkorovainy, A., and Murphy, B.E.P. 1973
    Isolation of cytoplasmic glucocorticoid-binding protein(s)
    from rat liver by means of affinity chromatography, and its
    partial characterization. *Biochim. Biophys. Acta* 328:133-144.

PROGESTERONE RECEPTORS OF CHICK OVIDUCT

William T. Schrader and Bert W. O'Malley

Department of Cell Biology
Baylor College of Medicine
Houston, TX 77030

ABSTRACT

The chick oviduct progesterone receptor has been purified to homogeneity by affinity chromatography and its molecular action studied *in vitro*. The native receptor is a 200,000 MW dimer of two dissimilar 4S subunits with different intranuclear function. The receptors directly regulate RNA chain initiation sites in oviduct chromatin by interactions involving target tissue nuclear acceptor sites. There is a 1:1 correspondence between receptor "acceptor" sites and RNA sites. Only the dimer form of the receptor is active *in vitro* on chromatin templates. The study suggests a novel model for hormone action which can be tested directly in this system.

INTRODUCTION

All steroid hormones thus far described have been found to bind to specific molecules termed receptor proteins. These proteins mediate hormone action by the steroid-receptor complex binding to the nuclear chromatin to regulate gene expression (O'Malley and Means, 1974). The processes involved in regulation have only recently come under direct experimental study in isolated systems. Although considerable information has been obtained about these

This research was supported by National Institutes of Health Grants HD-8188, HD-7857, HD-7495 and by a Ford Foundation Grant to the Cell Biology Department, Baylor College of Medicine.

molecules, the issue has been somewhat clouded by the difficulties
of working with unstable proteins present in low concentrations
(about 10^{-9} M) (Jensen and DeSombre, 1974). Secondly, the receptors appear to undergo molecular associations with each other of a
complicated nature not easily understood by the prevailing technique of sucrose-gradient ultracentrifugation (Notides, 1975).

It appears that all steroid receptors share a set of general
molecular parameters which makes experiments in one system easier
to fit into the framework of studies in another system. The first
of these similarities is a change in sedimentation constant with
both temperature and ionic strength (Erdos, 1970; Jensen, Numata,
Brecher, and DeSombre, 1971). Receptor monomers sediment at about
4S, and associate with each other to form dimers or higher aggregates (Schrader, Heuer, and O'Malley, 1975). In the rat uterus,
this dimerization has been termed "activation;" estrogen receptor
monomers undergo a shift in sedimentation coefficient from 4S to
about 5.4S, corresponding to an increase in molecular weight from
70,000 to 130,000 (Notides, 1975). Because of the use of crude
preparations for these studies, the sedimentation values can be
misleading and are subject to variation due to association with
polyanions (Chamness and McGuire, 1974) and by other proteins in
the extract (Stancel and Gorski, 1973).

In studies of progesterone action in chick oviduct, these
events have also been observed (Buller, Toft, Schrader, and O'Malley, 1975; Sherman, Corvol, and O'Malley, 1970). The 4S units are
highly asymmetric proteins with molecular weights of about 100,000.
They behave anomalously in sucrose gradients due to this asymmetry.
A number of their properties have been determined; the receptors
are now believed to function as dimers (6S) of two dissimilar subunits which have been isolated independently and shown to differ
with respect to their size, charge, and nuclear function (Buller,
Schwartz, Schrader, and O'Malley, 1976; Schrader and O'Malley,
1972; Schrader, Toft, and O'Malley, 1972).

The mechanism of steroid hormone action may be related to the
distinctive properties of this 6S progesterone receptor dimer
(O'Malley, Spelsberg, Schrader, Chytil, and Steggles, 1972;
Schrader et al., 1975). The dimer binds to nuclei and chromatin
but not to DNA. It is composed of A and B subunits which have
different and unique properties. The B subunit binds to the nonhistone protein-DNA complexes of oviduct chromatin but not to pure
DNA, while the A subunit binds to pure DNA, but poorly to chromatin (O'Malley et al., 1972; Schrader et al., 1972). Accordingly,
these observations have led to the suggestion that the A subunit
could be the actual gene regulatory protein and the B subunit
could specify where the A protein is to localize (O'Malley et al.,
1972; Schrader et al., 1975). In the absence of the B component of
the dimers, the A subunit alone should encounter difficulty in local-

izing the specific initiation sites (genes) it is to regulate, while the B subunit alone should be totally inactive as a transcriptional stimulant.

The chick oviduct provides an excellent model system for the hormonal control of cellular gene expression. Chronic administration of estrogen over a period of 10-14 days results in growth and differentiation of the chick oviduct, involving significant alterations in gene transcription.

Recent studies have demonstrated increased transcription of unique sequence DNA during oviduct growth (Liarakos, Rosen, and O'Malley, 1973), increased levels of nuclear RNA (O'Malley and McGuire, 1968), increased RNA polymerase activity (Cox, Haines, and Carey, 1973; O'Malley, McGuire, Kohler, and Korenman, 1969) enhanced chromatin template capacity, and changes in chromatin non-histone proteins (Spelsberg, Steggles, Chytil, and O'Malley, 1973). Preceding the well documented specific changes in protein synthesis (Comstock, Rosenfeld, O'Malley, and Means, 1972; Means, Comstock, Rosenfeld, and O'Malley, 1972; Rosenfeld, Comstock, Means, and O'Malley, 1972), there was an unequivocal net accumulation of specific, biologically active messenger RNA coding for ovalbumin (Chan, Means, and O'Malley, 1973; Harris, Rosen, Means, and O'Malley, 1975; Palmiter and Smith, 1973). When estrogen treatment of the chicks is discontinued, a reduction in the overall level of RNA and protein synthesis occurs and the cell's ability to synthesize specific proteins such as ovalbumin decreases (Chan *et al.*, 1973; Palmiter, 1973). After 12 days of hormone withdrawal the rate of ovalbumin biosynthesis is less than 1% of that observed in hormonally stimulated chicks (Harris *et al.*, 1975). If either estrogen or progesterone is readministered (secondary stimulation) there is a rapid increase in the production of ovalbumin mRNA and the induction of the other egg white proteins begins again (Palmiter, 1973). Therefore, the chick oviduct provides a system to study a specific endocrine response in which overall gene expression can be dramatically altered while a specific marker for measuring changes in the transcription rate of a single gene is available.

Because of the central role of receptors in dictating hormone responses, it was essential to have available homogeneous receptor preparations. These preparations could then be used in cell-free reconstitution studies for further investigations of the process by which steroid hormones alter differential gene expression. We, therefore, undertook purification and characterization of the chick oviduct progesterone receptor.

This chapter discusses receptor characterization in the chick oviduct system. However, the methods are generally applicable to any receptor system. The central difference among receptors for steroid hormones seems to be the half-life of the hormone-receptor complex; the behavior of the complexes is similar in all systems.

MATERIALS AND METHODS

Preparation of Crude Cytoplasmic Receptors

The standard buffer used is 10 mM Tris HCl, pH 7.4, containing 1 mM Na_2EDTA and 12 mM 1-thioglycerol (Buffer A). This is supplemented with various amounts of KCl as indicated below. Oviducts are cut from chicks freshly killed by cervical dislocation and are obtained by a ventral incision. The oviducts are clipped free of mesentery, blotted, rinsed in ice-cold 0.9% NaCl saline solution and homogenized using a Polytron (Brinkmann Instruments, PT-10).

It is important to maintain the solution at 0° C. The crude homogenate is then centrifuged in a swinging-bucket rotor (Sorvall HB-4) for 10 minutes at 10,000 rpm. The layer of floating lipid is drawn off and the crude low-speed cytoplasmic material decanted. The low-speed supernatant fraction is then centrifuged at 150,000 xg for 1 hour in a Spinco swinging-bucket rotor to prepare the cytosol. Another small lipid plug is found after this centrifugation, and is carefully drawn off by aspiration.

One ml of cytosol prepared as described above contains about 20 mg of protein and will contain about 10 nmoles of progesterone receptor sites. This is about 7 ng of steroid bound at saturation or 2×10^6 dpm of ^3H progesterone at 50 Ci/mmole.

Ammonium Sulfate Precipitation

The crude cytosol receptor preparation can be purified 20- to 30-fold in about 70%-80% yield by precipitation of the receptors at 30% saturation of ammonium sulfate. Saturated ammonium sulfate, neutralized with NH_4OH, is prepared in Buffer A and added drop-wise to stirred cytosol in ice until the final solution is 30% saturated in ammonium sulfate. The solution turns cloudy but not opaque, and rigorous removal of lipid during the preparation of the cytosol results in much less visible precipitate at this step. After 30 minutes the white precipitate is collected by centrifugation in a Sorvall HB-4 rotor at 10,000 rpm for 20 minutes. The use of the swinging-bucket rotor enhances recovery and provides a small, compact pellet. The straw-colored supernatant fraction contains any free steroid as well as corticosteroid binding globulin (CBG) and a small quantity of the progesterone receptor protein. Some yield is sacrificed at this step to exclude recovery of CBG in the pellet. This method can be used to precipitate either progesterone-receptor

complex or the nascent, uncomplexed receptors. The tubes containing the pellets are kept rigorously cold, and the inside walls
above the pellet rinsed under a stream of cold H_2O, after which
the walls are wiped dry.

The receptor pellets are redissolved in cold Buffer A. After
about 30 minutes the denatured material is removed by brief centrifugation. Hormone in the supernatant consists of about 95% receptor complex, with only a small amount of free steroid. Hence, this
technique has the added advantage of preparing receptors free of
unbound ligand (Buller *et al.*, 1975).

Ion-exchange Chromatography

DEAE cellulose ion exchange chromatography used Whatman DE-52
ion exchange resin prepared in 10 mM Tris buffer containing 1 mM
EDTA and 12 mM 1-thioglycerol. The resin (Whatman DE-52) was washed and equilibrated in Buffer A. A 10 ml column of DEAE cellulose
was prepared in a 50 ml plastic syringe. Millipore glass prefilt-
ers or stainless steel screen were used above and below the resin.
The columns were equilibrated in buffer; then cytosol or an ammonium sulfate precipitate was applied to the column; free progesterone, unlike estradiol, does not bind to DEAE cellulose. The column
was washed with buffer and the receptors eluted using a KCl gradient (0 to 0.4 M KCl).

At the analytical scale, columns of phosphocellulose made from
Whatman P-11 were prepared in 10 mM Tris buffer at pH 7.4. A typical column size of 5 ml packed volume has adequate capacity to
chromatograph the receptors from about 5 g of tissue. Receptors
were applied in low ionic strength and again chromatographed either
by stepwise or by gradient elution using KCl. The receptor subunits
bind somewhat more tightly to phosphocellulose than they do to DEAE
cellulose and consequently they are eluted from the column between
0.2 and 0.4 M KCl.

Progesterone receptors will adsorb readily to hydroxylapatite
equilibrated in 0.01 M phosphate buffer at pH 7.4. The hydroxylapatite column was loaded with receptors in a Tris buffer solution
containing up to 1 M KCl. The column was washed free of KCl and
then was eluted subsequently using a potassium phosphate gradient
from 0 to 0.3 M.

Steroid-affinity Chromatography

Chick oviduct progesterone receptors were quantitatively removed from the ammonium sulfate precipitate by a column of deoxy-
corticosterone-21-hemisuccinate attached to Sepharose beads through

a denatured bovine serum albumin backbone. The steroid-hemisuccin-
ate derivative was coupled to the Sepharose at a final concentration of 1-2 μmoles per packed ml of gel. Nascent progesterone receptors from 20 g of tissue adsorb to a 1 ml column of this material (Kuhn, Schrader, Smith, and O'Malley, 1975).

        The column was washed with buffer containing 0.4 M KCl with-
out eluting the receptor. Other proteins with relatively little
affinity for the steroid passed directly through the column. The
column was then incubated with ^{3}H-progesterone for 1 hour at room
temperature. The column was next washed to collect the receptor
proteins released into solution. The first 1 ml of wash was applied to a 10 cm Sephadex G-75 column, which separated free hormone from that bound to macromolecules. The void volume of this
column contained labeled progesterone bound to receptor protein
(10^{-8} M). The entire process takes about 1.5 working days. Purification on the order of several thousand-fold was accomplished in
a single step.

        Recovered material was purified over 2000-fold. Early esti-
mates of receptor concentration in chick oviduct suggested that
they comprise 0.02% of the total protein present in a 105,000 xg
cytosol preparation. Thus, a 5000-fold purification would be required to achieve homogeneity. The material eluted from the affinity column would, therefore, be 40%-50% pure. Polyacrylamide
gel electrophoresis in the presence of 1% sodium dodecyl sulfate
(SDS) revealed the presence of at least five protein bands. Two
of these bands have been shown to correspond to receptor components A and B.

        Final purification to homogeneity required chromatography on
a short DEAE-Sephadex column. Gradient elution with KCl (0-0.4 M
KCl) yielded a broad peak of bound ^{3}H-progesterone eluting at 0.25
M which was exclusively receptor protein free of all other proteins.

                                RESULTS

        We have described the behavior of progesterone receptors and
their aggregates in an earlier publication (Schrader et al., 1975).
The elution of labeled cytosol receptors on DEAE columns revealed a
complex pattern (Figure 1). The intact material behaved differently from the appearance of profiles obtained for receptors dissociated into their subunits by ammonium sulfate precipitation (Schrader
and O'Malley, 1972). After such a precipitation, subunit A elutes
at 0.1 or 0.15 M KCl and subunit B elutes at 0.2 M KCl on DEAE
columns.

        As shown in Figure 1, cytosol receptors yield very little free
A protein; most of the radioactivity elutes as a complex peak at

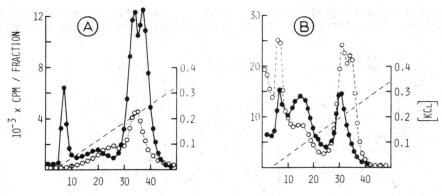

Figure 1. *DEAE cellulose elution profiles of unfractionated cyto-*
sol receptor-hormone complexes and dissociated subunits.
Columns (5 ml) were eluted with linear KCl gradients in
Buffer A. Panel A: Elution of labeled cytosol (●——●)
compared to elution profile of 30% saturated ammonium
sulfate precipitate (O---O) made from an equivalent
volume of cytosol. Panel B: Elution of labeled cyto-
sol (O---O) or of a dialyzed cytosol preparation of
equivalent volume (●——●). KCl concentrations deter-
mined by conductivity (----).

0.2-0.23 M. By sucrose-gradient ultracentrifugation and phosphocellulose chromatography (Schrader *et al.*, 1975), we found that
the 0.2 M KCl peak consisted of 6S receptor dimers, while the 0.23
M KCl peak was 8S material, consisting of higher aggregates.

Ammonium sulfate precipitation (30% saturation) yielded the
receptor subunits chromatographing as shown by the open circles in
Figure 1A. The yield was only about 50% of the total receptors in
cytosol. The shoulder at 0.15 M KCl was receptor A, separated
from the peak at 0.2 M of receptor B subunit.

Extensive dialysis of cytosol also converted receptors to subunits as shown in Figure 1B by the solid circles. In this case
the A protein eluted at 0.1 M KCl (A_1). Rechromatography showed
that the 0.1 M form produced by dialysis was clearly separable from
the 0.15 M KCl form seen upon ammonium sulfate precipitation at 30%
saturation (A_2).

The ammonium sulfate precipitate was shown to consist of equi-
molar amounts of A and B by chromatography of the redissolved
precipitate on DEAE, phosphocellulose and hydroxylapatite (Figure
2). The peak heights are nearly identical in all three cases.
Assignment of subunit identities to the peaks in this figure was

made by rechromatography of each peak on the other types of column
material. No interconversion of A and B has ever been detected.

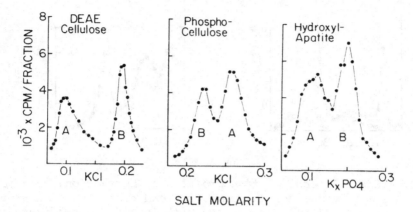

*Figure 2.   Resolution of receptor subunits A and B in equal amounts
by column chromatography using gradient elution. A 30%
ammonium sulfate cut of receptors was applied to either
DEAE cellulose (left panel), phosphocellulose (center
panel), or hydroxylapatite (right panel).*

*Table 1.   STEROID AFFINITY CHROMATOGRAPHY OF CHICK PROGESTERONE
RECEPTORS*

Step	Total protein[a] (mg)	Total receptor sites[b] (10^{-6} x dpm)	Specific activity[c] dpm/mg (x 10^{-6})	Yield (%)	Purification (-fold)
Cytosol	2788	185	0.066	100	1 x
30% pel- let	25.2	45.1	1.79	24	27
Affinity eluate	0.19	27.1	142.5	14.6	2150
DEAE-Seph- adex	0.052	13.6	200	8	4050

[a]Protein determined by method of Lowry *et al.*, 1951.

[b]Receptor sites determined by Scatchard plot, or by total dpm
of progesterone bound in affinity resin eluate as determined
by gel filtration.

[c]Theoretical maximum specific activity estimated at 10 dpm/mg.

From Kuhn *et al.*, 1975.

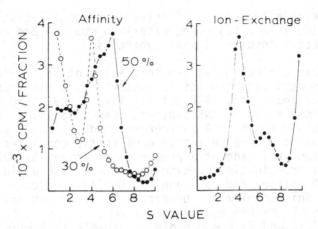

Figure 3. Sucrose gradient ultracentrifugation of receptors in an SW-50.1 rotor for 16 hours at 45,000 rpm. Left panel: Purified receptors made by steroid affinity chromatography. Before the affinity step cytosol was brought to either 30% (0---0) or 50% (●---●) saturation in ammonium sulfate to precipitate receptors as either monomers (4S) or intact dimers (6S), respectively. Right panel: Receptors purified (20% pure) by ion-exchange stepwise elutions showing both 4S and 6S forms present.

The methods for purification by affinity chromatography have already been published. As shown in Table 1, the material is highly purified and approaches the maximum theoretical specific activity (10^9 dpm/mg). This material was prepared by precipitation of cytosol at 30% ammonium sulfate. If 50% saturation was used, the results of Figure 3 were obtained. The left panel of Figure 3 shows that at 30%, the subunits recovered from the column ran at 4S. If 50% saturation was used, the affinity eluate sedimented as intact, 6S dimers.

The right-hand panel of Figure 3 shows a sucrose gradient profile of partially-purified (20% pure) receptors made by ion-exchange chromatography; some intact 6S dimer was also obtained by these procedures.

The capacity of oviduct chromatin to serve as a template for *E. coli* RNA polymerase has previously been shown to increase following estrogen administration to the immature chick (Cox, 1973; Spelsberg *et al.*, 1973). While chromatin template activity measurements may generally reflect the amount of DNA sequences made available to RNA polymerase, the components of such a reaction are so complex that these experiments shed little light on the biochemical mechanisms of hormone-induced alterations in gene transcription. In

order to determine the effect of esteogen on gene transcription in
the chick oviduct it appeared necessary to monitor and control all
of the parameters involved in RNA synthesis.

Procedures for measuring the initiation of RNA chains *in
vitro* were adopted from studies in bacterial and bacteriophage
systems (Bautz and Bautz, 1970: Lill, Lill, Sippel, and Hartmann,
1970). The initiation of RNA synthesis can be divided into two
basic processes. First, RNA polymerase binds randomly and reversibility to DNA to form a series of nonspecific complexes. However,
after sufficient time and at a proper temperature RNA polymerase
proximal to a true initiation site may form a stable binary complex with DNA (Sippel and Hartmann, 1970; Zillig, Zechel, and Rabussay, 1970). This complex has undergone a transition involving the
local opening of the DNA duplex structure (Travers, Baillie, and
Pedersen, 1973), and is now capable of rapidly initiating an RNA
chain (Hinkle and Chamberlin, 1972). The second process is the
actual initiation step in which RNA polymerase catalyzes the formation of the first phosphodiester bond between two nucleoside tri-
phosphates. By adding increasing amounts of RNA polymerase to a
fixed amount of template, the total number of available initiation
sites can be determined from the saturation level of RNA synthesis.

The number of initiation sites in estrogen-treated oviduct
chromatin was analyzed in an identical procedure. Chromatin (5 μg)
was preincubated for 30 minutes with increasing amounts of RNA
polymerase. Then RNA synthesis was started by the combined addition of nucleotides, rifampicin, and heparin. Heparin was added
to inhibit any contaminating RNase activity which, if present,
would decrease the average chain length of the RNA product (Cox,
1973; Tsai, Schwartz, Tsai, and O'Malley, 1975). The number of
initiation sites found after preincubation with RNA polymerase at
37° C was calculated to be 33,700/mg of DNA (based on a RNA number average chain length of 750 nucleotides and a base composition
of 25% UMP). These data correspond to one initiation site per
26,000 base pairs of DNA. Thus, chromatin contains only about 2%
of the total initiation sites found in deproteinized DNA.

Although incapable of inducing egg white protein synthesis in
the oviduct during primary stimulation, progesterone not only re-
establishes ovalbumin protein synthesis but appears generally to
mimic estrogen as a secondary stimulant to hormonally withdrawn
chicks (McKnight, Pennequin, and Schimke, 1975; Palmiter, 1973).
Furthermore, the similarity in the extent of egg white protein
synthesis induced by progesterone suggests that the time course of
induction of RNA synthesis during secondary stimulation is similar
to estrogen and not influenced by the cytodifferentiation of new
tubular gland cells (Palmiter, 1973). In order to test progesterone receptors *in vitro*, we wished to adopt a system in which progesterone had a large effect upon chromatin transcription *in vivo*.

We chose first to determine progesterone's effect using the rifampicin assay.

Estrogen-treated chicks were withdrawn from hormone treatment
for 12 days and then restimulated with a single injection of progesterone (2.0 mg). Oviduct chromatin was isolated from these
chicks and assayed by the rifampicin-challenge technique. The
number of initiated RNA chains was calculated as described above.
As shown in Table 2, withdrawn chromatin had a capacity to support
the initiation of 8,100 RNA chains/pg of DNA. Following a single
injection of progesterone, a rapid increase in the number of initiation sites was found. Within a half-hour of hormone treatment the
number of initiation sites had nearly doubled to a level of 16,800
sites. After one hour of progesterone stimulation a maximum of
23,600 initiation sites was detected. Thereafter, the number of
initiation sites declined so that by 24 hours after progesterone
administration, 13,800 sites were observed. Thus, progesterone
mimics estrogen action at the molecular level in the withdrawn
chick oviduct.

Since an increase in RNA chain initiation sites was detected
within 30 minutes of progesterone administration to withdrawn
chicks these results appeared to be consistent with our hypothesis
that steroid receptor complexes enter target cell nuclei and modu-
late gene transcription. Nevertheless, there has previously been
no proof that the steroid receptor complex could act directly on
nuclear chromatin to stimulate transcription. Toward this end, we
tested the effect of purified progesterone receptor complexes on
all parameters of transcription using a reconstituted cell-free
system which contained the following purified components: proges-

Table 2.   *EFFECT OF PROGESTERONE ON RNA INITIATION SITES
IN WITHDRAWN OVIDUCT CHROMATIN IN VIVO PROG -
IN VITRO SITE ASSAY*

Time after injection (hr)	Initiation sites per pg chromatin DNA
0	8,100
0.5	16,800
1	23,600
2	16,400
6	14,200
24	13,800

12 days DES-10 days withdrawn
Initial Elongation Rate: 8 nucleotides/sec.
Number Average Chain Size: 750 nucleotides

terone receptor complex, *E. coli* RNA polymerase, ribonucleotides, cofactors, and chromatin from withdrawn chicks (Schwartz, Kuhn, Buller, Schrader, and O'Malley, 1976).

A fixed concentration of withdrawn oviduct chromatin (5 µg) was preincubated with increasing quantities of purified progesterone receptor complex (up to 1 x 10^{-8}M) for 30 minutes at 22° C. The cytoplasmic progesterone receptor complex contains mainly 6S dimers of A (80,000 MW) and B (117,000 MW) subunits and was purified over 2000-fold by the affinity chromatography procedure of Kuhn *et al*. (1975). The chromatin receptor complexes were next incubated for an additional 30 minutes with a saturating concentration of RNA polymerase (15 µg) to allow for the formation of stable initiation complexes. Finally, rifampicin and nucleotides were added, as before, for a 15-minute RNA synthesis period. RNA synthesis, in the presence of rifampicin, increased in a receptor dose-dependent manner in which the half-maximal stimulation occurred at a progesterone receptor concentration of 0.5 x 10^{-8}M (Figure 4). In this experiment, RNA synthesis was stimulated to a

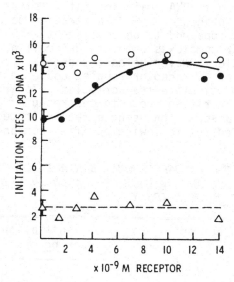

Figure 4.   Tissue-specific stimulation of chromatin RNA chain initiation sites in vitro by purified receptor 6S complexes. Initiations in 5 µg each of several chromatins were measured using the rifampicin-challenge assay and 15 µg of E. coli RNA polymerase. Purified receptors (affinity column eluate) were about 25% pure. Receptor molarity assumes 1 progesterone/100,000 MW unit. Addition of receptors to oviduct (●——●), liver (O---O), or erythrocyte (∆---∆) at indicated molarities. From Schwartz et al., 1976.

maximum of 62% over control values at 1.0×10^{-8}M of progesterone receptor complex.

We tested the sensitivity of the receptor stimulation to various inhibitors. We found that RNA synthesized in the presence of receptor and chromatin was completely dependent upon template and inhibited by actinomycin D. Furthermore, none of the components alone contained significant synthetic activity and, hence, neither the chromatin, polymerase, nor receptor were contaminated with other enzymes which were capable of incorporating [^{3}H]UTP into acid insoluble material. With the addition of α-amaitin, a potent inhibitor of uekaryotic RNA polymerase II, there was little effect on the progesterone-receptor directed stimulation of RNA transcription. These data showed that the stimulation of RNA synthesis was not due to the activation of endogenous RNA polymerase, which could have been a contaminant in chromatin preparations, but rather was due to transcription by the added *E. coli* enzyme. Identical results were obtained in other experiments using chick oviduct RNA polymerase II (Schwartz *et al.*, 1976). Moreover, the study showed that the increased RNA synthesis was dependent upon the native structure of the hormone-receptor complex since neither free progesterone nor boiled receptor was effective in stimulating RNA synthesis.

Quantitation of RNA initiation sites induced by receptor steroid complexes was determined by measuring the total incorporation of nucleotides in the presence of rifampcin divided by the average chain length number of the RNA product. We calculated that withdrawn chromatin in this experiment had the capacity to code for 10,000 RNA chains per pg of DNA. After an *in vitro* incubation with progesterone-receptor complexes, the capacity to initiate RNA synthesis increased to 15,200 sites at 1×10^{-8}M receptor. There were no significant differences in either the size of the RNA product or in the initial rate of elongation. Thus, the purified receptor preparation had stimulated the RNA initiation events, rather than elongation steps.

The kinetics for the stimulation of chromatin transcription *in vitro* revealed a $T_{1/2}$ of 15 minutes (Schwartz *et al.*, 1976). This value is close to the optimal time for receptor binding to chromatin at 22° C and similar to the kinetics of receptor appearance in nuclei *in vivo* and *in vitro* following progesterone administration (Buller *et al.*, 1975; O'Malley, Sherman, Toft, Spelsberg, Schrader, and Steggles, 1971). A maximal increase in transcription was found to occur within 30 minutes after the addition of receptor. Previous studies have demonstrated a quantitative tissue specificity for binding of oviduct progesterone receptor complexes to nuclei and to chromatin (Buller *et al.*, 1975; Jaffe, Socher, and O'Malley, 1975). It was, therefore, of interest to investigate the ability of the receptor to modify the transcriptional response of various chromatins and DNA.

At receptor concentrations which produced maximal stimulation there were 3,700 initiation sites per pg of DNA in oviduct chromatin but only 750 and 300 additional receptor-induced sites in liver and erythrocyte chromatin, respectively (Figure 4). Thus, it appears that the progesterone receptor-mediated effect is at least partly dependent on the presence of tissue specific proteins in the oviduct chromatin. These proteins may be related to the nonhistone chromosomal proteins, which convey quantitative tissue specificity for receptor binding and comprise a vital part of the chromatin "acceptor sites" for steroid hormone-receptor binding (Spelsberg *et al.*, 1972; Spelsberg, Steggles, and O'Malley, 1971).

The data presented above strongly support our proposal that direct transcriptional control is the primary locus of steroid hormone action. Since progesterone can induce ovalbumin in withdrawn chicks, it was conceivable that the purified progesterone receptors could induce the ovalbumin gene in isolated oviduct chromatin. Such a demonstration would strongly reaffirm the notion that the *in vitro* receptor-chromatin interaction mimics the events *in vivo*. To test this we transcribed oviduct chromatin *in vitro* in the presence of bacterial RNA polymerase. The RNA synthesized was isolated and reacted with [^{3}H]DNA complementary to ovalbumin mRNA (cDNA$_{ov}$; Harris *et al.*, 1975). The tritiated cDNA$_{ov}$ hybridization to mRNA$_{ov}$ sequences in the RNA samples constituted a specific probe to estimate the concentration of these sequences. Briefly, a fixed concentration of [^{3}H]cDNA$_{ov}$ is allowed to hybridize with an excess of either pure mRNA$_{ov}$ standards or with RNA synthesized *in vitro*. From the kinetics of the cDNA$_{ov}$-mRNA$_{ov}$ reassociation reaction at various RNA concentrations, the mRNA$_{ov}$ concentration in the extract can be determined.

When RNA synthesized from oviduct chromatin was tested using this assay mRNA$_{ov}$ was indeed synthesized *in vitro* (Harris, Schwartz Tsai, Roy, and O'Malley, 1976). Ovalbumin mRNA synthesis required addition of RNA polymerase and was only detected in the chromatin prepared from estrogen-stimulated oviducts. These results implied that the ovalbumin gene in chromatin is accessible to RNA polymerase during hormone stimulation, but is inaccessible or "repressed" prior to hormone administration and following hormone withdrawal (Harris *et al.*, 1976).

Using this approach, we then asked whether the purified progesterone receptor complex could directly stimulate the transcription of the ovalbumin gene in a cell-free system as shown in Table 3. Bulk amounts of RNA were synthesized from both control-withdrawn chromatin and from chromatin incubated in the presence of progesterone receptor (1×10^{-8} M). Both RNA preparations were assayed for complementary sequences to [^{3}H]cDNA$_{ov}$. The RNA synthe-

Table 3.   *IN VITRO SYNTHESIS OF OVALBUMIN mRNA FROM CHICK OVIDUCT*
           CHROMATIN

Source of chromatin	Proges- terone receptor $(1 \times 10^{-8} M)$	Chromatin in reac- tion $(\mu g \; DNA)$	RNA synthe- sized (μg)	Percent $mRNA_{OV}$ in RNA	pg $mRNA$ syn- thesized $(\times 10^{-3})$	pg $mRNA_{OV}$ per μg DNA
With- drawn ovi- duct	−	400	125	0.0015	1.9	0-4.8
With- drawn ovi- duct	+	400	135	0.0015	20.0	50.0

Chromatin was preincubated with progesterone receptor for
30 min. at 22° C. Bulk RNA synthesis was performed at 22°
C, as described by Chang *et al.*, 1976. The purified RNA
was hybridized with $cNDA_{OV}$ (1.5 µg) as described previously (Harris *et al.*, 1975).

sized in the presence of receptor-hormone complex contained a 10-
fold enrichment of $mRNA_{OV}$ sequence as compared to that found in un-
treated withdrawn chromatin controls. It, thus, appears that a
steroid-receptor complex may act directly on chromatin to enhance
the number of initiation sites for RNA synthesis; leading to the
synthesis of specific mRNA for induced proteins.

We discussed above the fact that the progesterone receptor
consists of two similar, but nonidentical, subunits (A and B) in
the form of a species which sedimented on (low salt) sucrose gradients at ∿6S. The studies of the *in vitro* effects of progesterone
receptor upon RNA chain initiation were carried out utilizing receptor preparations which contained large amounts of the 6S receptor dimer species. We undertook an evaluation of the effects of
the receptor subunits individually. If, as we postulated, the A
subunit is truly a regulatory protein, it might be expected to alter transcription, but to do so less efficiently than the intact
dimer. Conversely, if the dimers B subunit is merely a specifier
protein which carries the A protein to the neighborhood of responsive genes, it should be ineffective in stimulating chromatin
transcription. We tested this concept by adding homogeneous A, B,
or partially purified 6S A·B dimer to chromatin prior to the transcription assay as shown in Figure 5. The intact 6S dimer was
again capable of stimulating RNA chain initiation at low concentra-

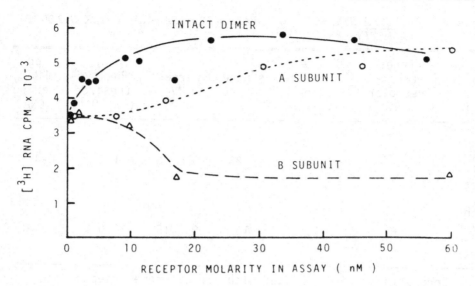

Figure 5. *Comparison of effectiveness of receptor dimers and sub-*
units in chromatin initiation site assay. Receptors
prepared by stepwise elution from ion-exchange columns.
Dimer (●——●), A subunit (O---O), and B subunit (Δ---Δ)
were tested individually in rifampicin-challenge assay.

tions. The isolated B subunit was ineffective in stimulating transcription from oviduct chromatin at any concentration tested. At
very high concentrations (10^{-7}M) inhibitory effects were often
noted. The isolated A subunit, on the other hand, was capable of
stimulating transcription, but only at significantly higher concentrations ($\sim$10-15-fold) than that required for the intact dimer.
Transcription experiments combining A and B together without recom-
bination showed no cooperative effect. Clearly, the 6S form is
necessary for optimal activity. These data support, but do not
yet prove, our hypothesis that the active form of the chick oviduct
progesterone receptor is a 6S dimer consisting of a specifier subunit (B) complexed with a regulatory subunit (A)(Buller *et al.*,
1976; O'Malley *et al.*, 1971; Schrader *et al.*, 1975).

DISCUSSION

The above data are consistent with the following model of
steroid hormone action which is presented in Figure 6. Steroids
enter target cells probably by passive diffusion and bind to cytoplasmic receptors. Under physiological salt conditions, the receptors consist of two subunits combined to form dimers sedimenting at 6S. The dimers can be reversibly dissociated, and are meta-

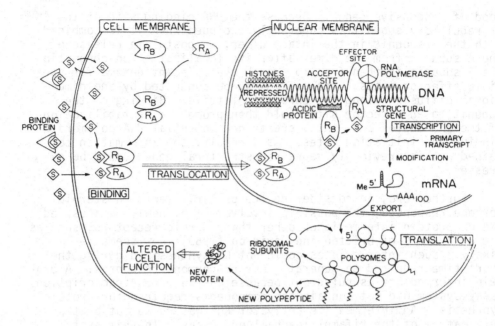

Figure 6.   A proposed model for steroid hormone action.

stable in the presence of hormone. They are present throughout
oviduct development and bind to nuclear acceptor sites with high
affinity ($K_d = 10^{-9}$ M) but do not bind to pure DNA when intact.

Two different subunit forms, A and B, make up the dimer: "A"
which binds only DNA and "B" which binds only chromatin. Both proteins are single polypeptide chains ($\sim$100,000 daltons) and sediment
at 4.2S. Each has one progesterone-binding site/molecule. The
hormone binding site can be distinguished from the site which binds
to the genome. Physiochemical experiments suggesting asymmetry of
the progesterone receptors have now been confirmed by electron
microscopy of purified receptor which shows it to be a prolate el-
lipsoid.

Following translocation to the cell nucleus, the receptor dimer binds through its B or specifier subunit to chromatin acceptor
sites consisting of DNA and chromatin-associated nonhistone proteins. This mechanism provides a concentration of active receptor
molecules in areas of the genome which are under hormonal control.
There is a requirement for two receptor-bound hormone molecules per
gene site; one on the B "specifier" subunit and one on the A "regulatory" subunit. The B subunit confers specificity at nuclear acceptor sites and, thereby, carries the A subunit to the neighbor-

hood of responsive genes. Because the DNA binding site of the A
or regulatory subunit is apparently occluded when it is combined
with the B subunit in the intact dimer, we postulate release of
the A subunit from the dimer after its localization on chromatin.
The A subunit is then free to search the adjacent genome for specific effector sites. The search may be conducted by one dimen-
sional diffusion along the chromatin lattice. Binding of the A
subunit to an effector site could then promote a destabilization
of the DNA duplex and, thus, create new potential RNA polymerase
binding and initiation sites. As a result, the information contained within previously repressed structural genes could be expressed.

Furthermore, in considering the primary events in steroid
hormone responses, the possible involvement of newly synthesized
RNA or protein intermediates other than steroid receptors, such as
the activators of Britten and Davidson (1969), now seems less
likely. Such intermediates could not be synthesized during the
short time required to generate *in vivo* hormone responses. A protein intermediate is ruled out because the *in vitro* transcription
assay system did not contain the components required for protein
synthesis. An intermediate activator RNA was ruled out by the
very nature of the rifampicin-challenge assay. In this system,
receptors and polymerase were incubated with chromatin in the absence of RNA synthesis. RNA synthesis was then started and further enzyme initiation was rapidly blocked by the addition of nucleotides, heparin, and rifampicin. The receptor-mediated increase
in the number of sites available for RNA chain initiation must
have occurred prior to all RNA synthesis, therefore, no functional
activator RNA's could have been generated.

In summary, the results presented in this manuscript are in-
consistent with models of steroid hormone action which postulate
a requirement for RNA or protein intermediates to be induced which
then exert secondary effects on transcription. Rather, the data
presented here support our proposal that direct, positive regulation of nuclear gene transcription is the mechanism of steroid
hormone action in eukaryotic cells.

REFERENCES

Bautz, E.K.F. and Bautz, F.A. (1970) Initiation of RNA synthesis:
    The function of σ in the binding of RNA polymerase to promoter
    sites. *Nature* 226:1219-1222.
Britten, R.J. and Davidson, E.H. (1969) Gene regulation for higher
    cells: A theory. *Science* 165:349-357.
Buller, R.E., Schwartz, R.J., Schrader, W.T., and O'Malley, B.W.
    (1976) Progesterone-binding components of chick oviduct: *In
    vitro* effect of receptor subunits on gene transcription. *J.*

Biol. Chem. 250:801-808.

Chan, L., Means, A.R., and O'Malley, B.W. (1973) Rates of induction of specific translatable messenger RNAs for ovalbumin and avidin by steroid hormones. *Proc. Nat'l. Acad. Sci. USA* 70:1870-1874.

Chamness, G.C. and McGuire, W.L. (1972) Estrogen receptor in the rat uterus. Physiological forms and artifacts. *Biochemistry* 11:2466-2472.

Comstock, J.P., Rosenfeld, G.C., O'Malley, B.W., and Means, A.R. (1972) Estrogen-induced changes in translation, and specific messenger RNA levels during oviduct differentiation. *Proc. Nat'l. Acad. Sci. USA* 69:2377-2380.

Cox, R.F. (1973) Transcription of high-molecular-weight RNA from hen-oviduct chromatin by bacterial and endogenous form-B RNA polymerases. *Eur. J. Biochem.* 39:49-61

Cox, R.F., Haines, M., & Carey, N. (1973) Modification of the template capacity of chick-oviduct chromatin for form-B RNA polymerase by estradiol. *Eur. J. Biochem.* 32, 513-524.

Cuatrecasas, P. and Anfinson, C.B. (1971) Affinity chromatography. *Ann. Rev. Biochem.* 40:259-278.

Edelman, I.S. and Fimognari, G.M. (1968) I. Modes of hormone action on the biochemical mechanism of action of aldosterone. *Rec. Progr. Horm. Res.* 24:1-44.

Erdos, T., Best-Belpomme, M., and Bessada, R. (1970) A rapid assay for binding estradiol to uterine receptor(s). *Anal. Biochem.* 37:244-252.

Fujii, T., and Villee, C.A. (1968) Effect of testosterone on ribonucleic acid metabolism in the prostate, seminal vesicle, liver and thymus of immature rats. *Endocrinology* 82:463-467.

Gorski, J. and Nicolette, W. (1963) Early estrogen effects on newly synthesized RNA and phospholipid in subcellular fractions of rat uteri. *Arch. Biochem. Biophys.* 103:418-423.

Hamilton, T.H., Widnell, C.C., and Tata, J.R. (1965) Sequential stimulation by oestrogen of nuclear RNA synthesis and DNA-dependent RNA polymerase activities in rat uterus. *Biochim. Biophys. Acta.* 108:168-172.

Harris, S.E., Rosen, J.M., Means, A.R., and O'Malley, B.W. (1975) Use of a specific probe for ovalbumin messenger RNA to quantitate estrogen-induced gene transcripts. *Biochemistry* 14:2072-2081.

Harris, S.E., Schwartz, R.J., Tsai, M.J., Roy, A.K., and O'Malley, B.W. (1976) Effect of estrogen on gene expression in the chick oviduct: *In vitro* transcription of the ovalbumin gene in chromatin. *J. Biol. Chem.* 251:524-529.

Hartman, H., Nonikel, K.O., Kniisel, F., and Niiesh, J. (1967) The specific inhibition of the DNA-directed RNA synthesis by rifamycin. *Biochim. Biophys. Acta.* 145:843-844

Hinkle, D.C. and Chamberlain, M.J. (1972) Studies of the binding of *Escherichia coli* RNA polymerase to DNA - I. The role of *sigma* subunit in site selection. *J. Mol. Biol.* 70:157-185.

Jaffe, R.C., Socher, S.H., and O'Malley, B.W. (1975) An analysis
    of the binding of the chick oviduct progesterone-receptor to
    chromatin. *Biochim. Biophys. Acta*. 399:403-419.
Jensen, E.V., Mohla, S., Gorell, T.A., and DeSombre, E.R. (1974)
    The role of estrophilin in estrogen action. *Vitamins and
    Hormones* 32:89-127.
Jensen, E.V., Numata, M., Brecher, P.I., and DeSombre, E.R. (1971)
    Hormone-receptor interaction as a guide to biochemical mecha-
    nism. *Biochem. Soc. Symp*. 32:133-159.
Kenney, F.T. and Kull, F.J. (1963) Hydrocortisone-stimulated syn-
    thesis of nuclear RNA in enzyme induction. *Proc. Nat'l. Acad.
    Sci. USA* 50:493-499
Kuhn, R.W., Schrader, W.T., Smith, R.G., and O'Malley, B.W. (1975)
    Progesterone binding components of chick oviduct - X. Purifi-
    cation by affinity chromatography. *J. Biol. Chem*. 250:4220-
    4228.
Liarakos, C.D., Rosen, J.M.,and O'Malley, B.W. (1973) Effect of
    estrogen on gene expression in the chick oviduct - II.
    Transcription of chick tritiated unique deoxyribonucleic acid
    as measured by hybridization in ribonucleic acid excess.
    Biochemistry 12:2809-2816.
Lill, H., Lill, U., Sippel, A., and Hartmann, G. (1970) In:
    Lepetit colloquium on RNA polymerase and transcription
    (Silvestri, L.G., ed.), p. 55, North Holland Publishing Co.,
    Amsterdam.
Lowry, O.H., Rosebrough, N.J., Farr, A.L., and Randall, R.J. (1951)
    Protein measurement with the Folin phenol reagent. *J. Biol.
    Chem*. 193:265.
Mainwaring, W.I.P., Wilce, P.A., and Smith, A.E. (1974) Studies
    on the form and synthesis of messenger ribonucleic acid in the
    rat ventral prostate gland, including its tissue-specific
    stimulation by androgens. *Biochem. J*. 137:531-524.
McKnight, S.G., Pennequin, P., and Schimke, R.J. (1975) Induction
    of ovalbumin mRNA sequences by estrogen and progesterone in
    chick oviduct as measured by hybridization to complementary
    DNA. *J. Biol. Chem*. 250:8105-8110.
Means, A.R., Comstock, J.P., Rosenfeld, G.C., and O'Malley, B.W.
    (1972) Ovalbumin messenger RNA of chick oviduct: Partial
    characterization, estrogen dependence, and translation *in
    vitro*. *Proc. Nat'l. Acad. Sci. USA* 69:1146-1150.
Norman, A.W. (1966) Vitamin D mediated synthesis of rapidly label-
    ed RNA from intestinal mucosa. *Biochem. Biophys. Res. Commun*.
    23:335-340.
Notides, A.C., Hamilton, D.E., and Auer, H.E. (1975) A kinetic
    analysis of the estrogen receptor transformation. *J. Biol.
    Chem*. 250:3945-3950.
O'Malley, B.W. and McGuire, W.L. (1968) Altered gene expression
    during differentiation: Population changes in hybridizable
    RNA after stimulation of the chick oviduct with oestrogen.
    Nature 218:1249-1251.

O'Malley, B.W., McGuire, W.L., Kohler, P.O.,and Koreman, S.G.
    (1969) Studies on the mechanism of steroid hormone regula-
    tion of synthesis of specific proteins. *Recent Progr. Hor-
    mone Res.* 25:105-160.
O'Malley, B.W. and Means, A.R. (1974) Female steroid hormones and
    target cell nuclei. *Science* 183:610-620.
O'Malley, B.W., Schrader, W.T., and Spelsberg, T.C. (1973) In:
    Receptors for reproductive hormones (O'Malley, B.W. and Means,
    A.R., eds.), pp. 174-196, Plenum Publishing Corp., New York.
O'Malley, B.W., Sherman, M.R., Toft, D.O., Spelsberg, T.C.,
    Schrader, W.T., and Steggles, A.W. (1971) A specific oviduct
    target-tissue receptor for progesterone. Identification,
    characterization, partial purification, intercompartmental
    transfer kinetics and specific interaction with the genome.
    In: *Adv. Biosci.*, Vol. 7 (Raspé, G., ed.), pp. 213-234,
    Pergamon Press, New York.
O'Malley, B.W., Spelsberg, T.C., Schrader, W.T., Chytil, F., and
    Steggles, A.W. (1972) Mechanisms of interaction of a hor-
    mone-receptor complex with a genome of a eukaryotic target
    cell. *Nature* 235:141-144.
Palmiter, R.D. (1973) Rate of ovalbumin messenger ribonucleic
    acid synthesis in the oviduct of estrogen-primed chicks. *J.
    Biol. Chem.* 248:6230-8260.
Palmiter, R.D. and Smith, L.T. (1973) Purification and transla-
    tion of ovalbumin, conalbumin, ovomucoid and lysozyme mes-
    senger-RNA. *Mol. Biol. Reports* 1:129-134.
Rosenfeld, G.C., Comstock, J.P., Means, W.R., and O'Malley, B.W.
    (1972) Estrogen-induced synthesis of ovalbumin messenger
    RNA and its translation in a cell-free system. *Biochem. Bio-
    phys. Res. Commun.* 46:1695-1703.
Rosner, W. and Bradlow, H.L. (1971) Purification of corticoster-
    oid-binding globulin from human plasma by affinity chromato-
    graphy. *J. Clin. Endocrinol. Metab.* 33:193-198.
Schrader, W.T. (1975) Methods for extraction and quantification
    of receptors. *Methods Enzymol.* 36:187-211.
Schrader, W.T., Buller, R.E., Kuhn, R.W., and O'Malley, B.W.
    (1974) Molecular mechanisms of steroid hormone action. *J.
    Steroid Biochem.* 5:989-999.
Schrader, W.T., Heuer, S.S., and O'Malley, B.W. (1975) Progester-
    one receptors of chick oviduct: Identification of 6S receptor
    dimers. *Biol. Reproduct.* 12:134-142.
Schrader, W.T. and O'Malley, B.W. (1972) Progesterone-binding
    components of chick oviduct - IV. Characterization of puri-
    fied subunits. *J. Biol. Chem.* 247:51-59.
Schrader, W.T., Toft, D.O., and O'Malley, B.W. (1972) Progesterone-
    binding protein of chick oviduct - VI. Interaction of purified
    progesterone-receptor components with nuclear constituents.
    J. Biol. Chem. 247:2401-2407.
Schwartz, R.J., Kuhn, R.W., Buller, R.E., Schrader, W.T., and
    O'Malley, B.W. (1976) Progesterone-binding components of

chick oviduct: *In vitro* effects of purified hormone-receptor
complexes on the initiation of RNA synthesis in chromatin. *J. Biol. Chem.* 251:5166-5177.

Schwartz, R.J. Tsai, M.J., Tsai, S.Y., and O'Malley, B.W. (1975)
Effect of estrogen on gene expression in the chick oviduct -
V. Changes in the number of RNA polymerase binding and initi-
ation sites in chromatin. *J. Biol. Chem.* 250:5175-5182.

Sekeris, C.E. and Lang, N. (1964) Induction of dopa-decarboxylase
activity by insect messenger RNA in an *in vitro* amino acid incorporating system from rat liver. *Life Sci.* 3:625-632.

Sherman, M.R., Corvol, P.L., and O'Malley, B.W. (1970) Progesterone-binding components of chick oviduct - I. Preliminary characterization of cytoplasmic components. *J. Biol. Chem.* 245:
6085-6096.

Sica, V., Parikh, I., Nola, E., Puca, G.A., and Cuatrecasas, P.
(1973) Affinity chromatography and the purification of
estrogen receptors. *J. Biol. Chem.* 248:6543-6558.

Sippel, A.E. and Hartmann, G.R. (1970) Rifampicin resistance of
RNA polymerase in the binary complex with DNA. *Eur. J. Biochem.* 16:152-157.

Spelsberg, T.C., Steggles, A.W., Chytil, F., and O'Malley, B.W.
(1972) Progesterone-binding components of chick-oviduct - V.
Exchange of progesterone-binding capacity from target to non-
target tissue chromatins. *J. Biol. Chem.* 247:1368-1374.

Spelsberg, T.C., Steggles, A.W., and O'Malley, B.W. (1971) Progesterone-binding components of chick-oviduct - III. Chromatin acceptor sites. *J. Biol. Chem.* 246:4188-4197.

Stancel, G.M., Leang, K.M.T., and Gorski, J. (1973) Estrogen receptors in the rat uterus. Relationship between cytoplasmic
and nuclear forms of the estrogen binding protein. *Biochemistry* 12:2137-2141.

Stohs, S.J., Zall, J.E., and DeLuca, H.F. (1967) Vitamin D stimulation of [^{3}H]orotic acid incorporation into ribonucleic acid
of rat intestinal mucosa. *Biochemistry* 6:1304-1310.

Travers, A., Baillie, D.L., and Pederson, S. (1973) Effect of DNA
conformation on ribosomal RNA synthesis *in vitro*. *Nature New
Biol.* 243:161-163.

Tsai, M.J., Schwartz, R.J., Tsai, S.Y., and O'Malley, B.W. (1975)
Effects of estrogen on gene expression in the chick oviduct -
IV. Initiation of RNA synthesis on DNA and chromatin. *J. Biol. Chem.* 250:5165-5174.

Umezawa, H., Mizuno, S., Uamasaki, H., and Hitta, K. (1968) Inhibition of DNA-dependent RNA synthesis by rifamycins. *J. Antibiotics* 21:234-236.

Zillig, W., Zechel, D., Rabussay, D., Schachne, M., Sethi, V.S.,
Palm, P., Heil, A., and Seifert, W. (1970) On the role of
different subunits of DNA-dependent RNA polymerase from *E.
coli* in the transcription process. *Cold Spring Harbor Symp.
Quant. Biol.* 35:47-58.

DISCUSSION FOLLOWING DR. SCHRADER'S TALK

Dr. Hechter
I have been witness to the development of this story since it
first began and I, for one, would like to express my admiration
for the progressive succession of major research achievements of
the O'Malley group. I think it is fair to say that those interested in hormone action have generally followed the concepts and
techniques of the biochemists, protein chemists, and molecular
biologists. It is clear from this presentation that endocrinology
has come a long way from that point in time, when endocrinologists
became "instant" molecular biologists by injecting actinomycin-D
and cycloheximide into hormone-treated animals. It is apparent
this pursuit of steroid hormone action provides lessons for biology
generally and contributes to our understanding of the central problem of gene regulation in eukaryotes.

My question concerns the steroid hormone, ecdysone, which acts
to control metamorphosis in insects. In metamorphosis, there is a
dramatic shift in gene expression: one set of genes is turned "on"
and another gene set is turned "off." The change in "gene program"
induced by ecdysone is inhibited by the juvenile hormone of insects.
Although there have been problems trying to fit ecdysone into the
general pattern of steroid hormone action, I understand that this
problem has now been resolved. Can one account for steroid action
to change a program of gene expression in terms of the model presented by Schrader? Schrader's elegant presentation illustrates
how the progesterone receptor controls the activity of specific
genes in oviduct chromatin which are "open" and are not repressed
by chromatin proteins. In the model shown, transcription is initiated when one of the subunits of the occupied receptor dimer is
directed to, and binds to, a stretch of "naked" DNA (not covered
by protein). The model serves to illustrate how a steroid hormone
induces changes in the activity of genes, which are already expressed, but leaves the question open why the "naked" DNA stretch-
es are not being "read-out" in the absence of the receptor subunit
and what it is that the subunit does when it binds to DNA which
serves to promote initiation.

However, the model does not help me to understand steroid action in differentiation and development, where the changes involve
the "derepression" of sets of genes. What are your thoughts about
steroid action in regard to the latter process?

Dr. Schrader
Thank you for your comments. Your point is well taken and I'd
like to clarify two points. First of all, the last diagram I showed is a conceptual model only. There is no evidence regarding the
accessibility of DNA in the nucleus, whether it is free in solu-

131

tion, whether it is covered with protein, or in what state it is.
I'd like to point out in that regard one calculation which people
frequently overlooked. If you calculate the volume of the nucleus
and the amount of DNA in there, the concentration of DNA in a eukaryotic nucleus is about 100 mg/ml. I don't know how many of you
have tried to make a DNA solution, but 100 mg/ml is not a solution,
and so the nature of the genetic material and its packaging is entirely unknown. In the oviduct, there are different genes being
turned on. When we withdraw hormonal support, this is a case of a
differentiated tissue which is being allowed to regress, but not
to dedifferentiate. So presumably the ovalbumin gene we're looking at in this case has already been converted by some differentiation process into a form which can then be stimulated in the future by steroid hormone. When we look at this case, we're not
looking at gene differentiation; the gene is all set to go as soon
as the right signal comes to it, and the hormone receptor somehow
allows the polymerase to enter or some action like that. The process is gene induction, which may be a completely different bag,
perhaps, from gene differentiation. Why does ecdysone turn on a
different set of genes one time and another set of genes some
other time? For example, you would think that estradiol ought to
shut off some genes. It's like playing an organ. You can change
the sound of the organ by pulling stops out, which you normally
do, or by pushing them in. The ecdysone case clearly is pulling
stops out and pushing stops in.

Dr. Lata
     With the availability of this material in such vast quanti-
ties. . .

Dr. Schrader
     Half-vast quantities.

Dr. Lata
     Half-vast quantities! It is now possible to do some of the
very fundamental studies, some of the islands that we bypassed in
all of this, concerning the specifics of steroid binding. We've
been really concentrating on the protein and have almost forgotten
that the steroid is there. The steroid is necessary to bring
about the receptor, but what is it doing there; in your analysis
of the UV curves, just as a very small step forward, did you do a
curve analysis? Is that progesterone chromophoric group sticking
into a hydrophobic or a polar region?

Dr. Schrader
     I tried to do that. I was just doing this in a Cary 118, and
to do that you've got to have the instruments set up to do differential recording with split cells. The problem is the following:
you cannot make large quantities of the apoprotein, which contains
no hormone; it's less stable. We can make small amounts of it. We

have not been able to make large quantities of the apoprotein and then add the hormone to do the study you're talking about. There is obviously a change. The hormone does a couple of things to the protein, to the dimer. One; it induces the chromatin binding site on the B subunit because the receptor dimer does not bind the chromatin without hormone. Two; very interestingly, the hormone regulates the metastability of the dimer. The dimer is much more stable as AB complex without hormone.

Dr. Lata
    Would you eliminate the possibility that, once the complex gets to the chromatin, the steroid may have some function such as, say, Paul T'so has suggested or at least his experiments suggest? It might at that time, then, do something with the DNA.

Dr. Schrader
    The changes in melt temperature of the DNA and whatnot, which Dr. T'so looked at a number of years ago, and which other people have found, occur at rather high concentrations of steroid; number one. Number two; the receptor occupancy, the receptor-hormone complex occupancy in the nucleus seems to occur only as long as the steroid is on the receptor protein. Once it comes off, it looks like it's rapidly metabolized and probably cleared. The "off" reaction of steroid hormones has really never been studied very carefully. And, take cycling rats, the rat spends half its time doing degradative work, spending only half of its time doing catabolic work.

Dr. Hechter
    In considering your experiments on oviduct chromatin, I should like to ask whether the concentration and/or pattern of electrolytes in the incubation medium serve to influence transcription. I refer to monovalent cations as well as bivalent cations. You will remember that after the effects of ecdysone to induce "puffing" patterns in giant chromosomes in insects were described, Kroeger at Zurich reported that he could induce "puffing" by altering the sodium:potassium ratio in the media. Kroeger's report that the pattern of electrolytes may be critical in transcriptional control remains an intriguing possibility which can now be "checked out" in the chick oviduct chromatin system.

Dr. Schrader
    First, if I'm not mistaken, Dr. Kroeger was able to show changes in the puffing patterns of the chromosomes but was never able to induce dopa-decarboxylase, I don't believe. As far as your second question, about the divalent cations, I can shed a little bit of light on that. We've never looked at the effect of calcium on transcription. *E. coli* RNA polymerase is a manganese-dependent enzyme, and we have done manganese curves, and in fact you can show a manganese optimum. We work at roughly the manganese optimum.

There is also a KCl dependence to the enzyme, which is not clear
whether there are KCl effects on the template or what. This is
done roughly at the optimal. Divalent calcium is a poor substi-
tute for manganese. As far as I know it has no effect on the
polymerase. We've done these reactions in a variety of buffers
without any big change. We have chelating agents in the buffer
and then surpass what the EDTA will chelate.

Calcium, in my hands, has no effect at all on purified receptors. There is a calcium-dependent protease, which has already
been described in the oviduct. There is a calcium-dependent protease, which is a nonreceptor element, which will bind to the receptor and will clip the receptor apart into a hormone-binding
fragment and a nonhormone-binding fragment, and it will act on
both subunits. That activity is entirely absent in homogeneous
material, and calcium has no detectable effect on the aggregation
state, the hormone-binding kinetics, the molecular weight, or anything else I've bothered to take a look at to date. And lastly,
there is no calcium in the transcription experiments. So we have
to conclude that the receptor, in the absence of calcium, is able
to induce gene activity in a completely cell-free experiment in
the absence of calcium. After it's been extracted in the EDTA and
prepared I'm told that it has very low titers of calcium. It takes
a couple of days to make it in EDTA-containing buffers. I don't
know how much there is.

Dr. Triano
There is information that uterine muscle adrenergic receptors
change under the influence of estrogen and progesterone during the
estrous cycle. This is demonstrated or has been worked with in St.
Louis with isolated tissue bath. Do you have any information as to
whether this is actual alteration of the receptors, a cooperative
hormonal effect, or if it's possibly a dimer receptor site?

Dr. Schrader
We've looked at the aggregation state of other receptors in
other systems and can observe the same sort of ion-exchange chrom-
atographic pattern that I showed here for all the other ones that
we've looked at. Whether or not a heteroduplex of a progesterone-
receptor type A subunit with an estrogen type B subunit or something like that could go on, has not yet been looked at. I can
add one other fact and that is: if you purify progesterone receptors with no hormone on them, you end up with a preparation which
will bind only progesterone and not any of the other steroids. So
at least in the chick oviduct which also contains estrogen receptors, androgen receptors, and glucocorticoid receptors, the progesterone receptor is different enough from these other ones that
by a series of ion exchange steps you end up with a preparation
which has none of the other receptors in it. I hope that answered
your question; I may have overlooked what you had in mind.

Dr. Triano
In addition to that, does anything in the androgen/estrogen receptor mechanism alter, such as in adrenergic response of *alpha* receptors which convert to *beta* receptors under the influence of progesterone or vice versa?

Dr. Schrader
No, I'm not aware of any of that.

Dr. Hechter
Let me ask one final, perhaps naive, question. To get RNA polymerase II activity you need manganese or very high concentrations of magnesium. And when you add manganese to chromatin the levels required are 1-3 mM. Now, if you go into the cell, whether the cytoplasm or the nucleoplasm and ask the question, where do these rather considerable concentrations of free manganese come from, the answer is we don't really know. Is a mechanism needed to scavenge the cell so that the metal is collected and delivered to the right spots in the nucleus to permit the synthesis of messenger RNA's?

Dr. Schrader
I don't know.

Dr. DeGroot
How many copies of the ovalbumin gene are there per cell?

Dr. Schrader
There is one copy of the gene per cell.

Dr. DeGroot
What does it mean that you increase the number of initiation sites? Does that mean that there are only two states of the cell, either it is transcribing or it isn't? In other words, does your percentage increase reflect cells that go from nothing to 100% activity?

Dr. Schrader
Ovalbumin is only one of what we think to be thousands of genes controlled by estrogen. We have two independent assays. One, we can ask what's the total number of genes which are turned on, that's the number of initiation sites we think. Let's say that's what that represents: there are 20,000 sites. Well, that doesn't tell you about any one individual gene, so we use the cDNA for ovalbumin message, to look at one out of these 20,000, and we see the same events going on for both, for the 20,000 and for the one. I guess what's confusing you is: how does a unique gene for ovalbumin produce 10 or 20 thousand copies of ovalbumin message per cell for ovalbumin, whereas a unique gene-like tryptophan oxygenase in the liver produces many fewer copies? And the answer is,

no one knows. There's a whole bunch of possible ways it could go
on. We have measured the rate of elongation of all these different RNA's, and they all seem to be elongated at roughly similar
rates. So you can't account for it *in vitro*, for example. The
ovalbumin gene doesn't get made any quicker than everything else
gets made so the regulation of accumulation has got to be an inter-
play between synthesis and degradation. That's something about
which very little is known. I'd like to point out something that
Saul Roseman at Johns Hopkins pointed out to me one time, and that
is the fact that there's only been about a thousand proteins ever
described. Here we're talking about 20,000 genes, but what are
the other 19,000 genes doing? Are they informational RNA's that
are working in the nucleus or what? Are they just other proteins
which are present in very small amounts about which nothing is
known? Well, we don't know.

Dr. Freed
     Do progesterone antagonists bind preferentially to either of
the subunits?

Dr. Schrader
     There are no good progesterone antagonists the way there are
antagonists, for example, for estradiol or even for glucocorticoids for that matter. The hormone binding specificity of both
subunits is the same; there is no detectable difference within
limits of experimental error. I'm asking myself the mental question, "Are both of those polypeptide chains the same?" Well,
they're not exactly the same length and they do different things,
but they're single polypeptide chains, so does that mean that the
steroid-binding site part of the gene, the part of the amino acid
that forms the active site for binding the hormone, for those two
genes, is it really the same polynucleotide sequence or not, and
that's not clear. Maybe the technique I'm using, the binding
kinetic data, is simply not good enough to look. The way to do
it is, very simply, you take the A protein and the B protein, you
do cyanogen bromide fragments, you make tryptic digests, you look
at the peptide maps, and you look to see whether or not all the
spots are the same. Answer -- don't know, I haven't done the
experiment yet.

IDENTIFICATION AND REGULATION OF β-ADRENERGIC RECEPTORS

Robert J. Lefkowitz

Department of Medicine and Biochemistry
Duke University Medical Center
Durham, NC 27710

INTRODUCTION

The receptor concept has been used for some time to explain the striking specificity of hormone and drug effects on tissues. However, it is only within the past few years that a direct experimental approach to the study of these cellular structures has become possible. Since about 1970 radioactively-labeled hormones and drugs have been used with increasing frequency for the purpose of direct identification of a wide variety of receptors for polypeptide hormones and neurotransmitters. By contrast, a variety of technical problems have hindered such direct identification of the membrane-bound adrenergic receptors for catecholamines. Quite recently, these technical problems have been overcome (Lefkowitz, 1975).

There appear to be two main types of receptors for catecholamines. These have been termed α and β (Ahlquist, 1948). Of these, in general, only the β-adrenergic receptors appeared to be associated with the stimulation of adenylate cyclase activity (Robison, Butcher, and Sutherland, 1971). The association of β-adrenergic receptors with adenylate cyclase has been demonstrated in several ways. First, the order of potency of catecholamines for stimulating adenylate cyclase activity is generally that characteristic of the β-adrenergic receptor: isoproterenol > epinephrine > norepinephrine. By contrast, α-adrenergic effects have been defined by a different order of potency: epinephrine ≥ norepinephrine ≫ isoproterenol (Ahlquist, 1948). Whereas, β-adrenergic antagonists competitively inhibit catecholamine stimulation of adenylate cyclase, α-adrenergic antagonists do not. There is also good evidence that most, if not all, physiological β-adrenergic effects are mediated

137

by cyclic AMP through the stimulation of adenylate cyclase (Lefkowitz, 1976) by β-adrenergic agonists.

Early efforts to investigate adenylate cyclase-coupled β-adrenergic receptors by direct binding methods were frustrated by the heterogeneity of the sites labeled with the radioligands employed. These early studies generally employed tritium-labeled β-adrenergic agonists such as [³H](±)isoproterenol or [³H](±)norepinephrine. Such ligands appear to bind not only to β-adrenergic receptors but also to a large number of nonspecific-binding sites, the physiological significance of which remain unclear (Cuatrecausas, Tell, Sica, Parikh, and Chang, 1974; Lefkowitz, 1975; Lefkowitz, Limbird, Mukherjee, and Caron, 1976; Lefkowitz, 1976). However, the use of high affinity radioactively-labeled β-adrenergic antagonists has permitted the identification of receptor sites in membranes from a wide variety of tissues which appeared to possess all the essential characteristics expected of the adenylate cyclase coupled β-adrenergic receptors (Lefkowitz, 1975; Lefkowitz, 1976; Lefkowitz *et al.*, 1976).

Identification of β-adrenergic Receptors by Radioligand Binding

To date several ligands have been used to identify directly β-adrenergic receptors by binding techniques. These are [³H](±) propranolol (Atlas, Steer, and Levitzki, 1974; Levitzki, Atlas, and Steer, 1974), ¹²⁵I(±)hydroxybenzypindolol (Aurbach, Fedak, Woodard, Palmer, Hauser, and Troxler, 1974; Brown, Rodbard, Fedak, Woodard, and Aurbach, 1976), and [³H](-)dihydroalprenolol (Lefkowitz, Mukherjee, Coverstone, and Caron, 1974; Mukherjee, Caron, Coverstone, and Lefkowitz, 1975). Results with the different ligands appear to be quite comparable, although somewhat higher "nonspecific" binding appears to be noted with the racemic propranolol. Our own group has extensively studied the β-adrenergic receptors with [³H](-) dihydroalprenolol. The material is catalytically reduced with tritium, thus saturating a double bond. The resulting material, (-)[³H]dihydroalprenolol, has biological activity identical to that of native (-)alprenolol (Mukherjee *et al.*, 1975; Mukherjee, Caron, Millikin, Lefkowitz, 1976). Its specific radioactivity is about 35 Ci/mmol. We have used this ligand to study the β-adrenergic-binding sites in a wide variety of mammalian (Alexander, Davis, and Lefkowitz, 1975; Alexander, Williams, and Lefkowitz, 1975; Williams, Jarett, and Lefkowitz, 1976; Williams, Snyderman, and Lefkowitz, 1976; Zatz, Kebabian, Romero, Lefkowitz, and Axelrod, 1976) and nonmammalian tissues (Lefkowitz *et al.*, 1974; Mukherjee *et al.*, 1975; Mukherjee *et al.*, 1976). Our most extensive studies, however, have been with membranes derived from frog erythrocytes. These cells contain a catecholamine-responsive adenylate cyclase system (Lefkowitz, 1974; Rosen, Erlichman, and Rosen, 1970). Binding of (-)[³H]dihydroalprenolol to sites in membrane fractions derived from these erythrocytes possess all the

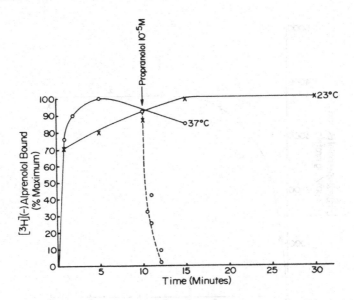

*Figure 1.   Forward and reverse kinetics of (-)[³H]dihydroalprenolol
binding to frog erythrocyte membranes.   This figure was
taken from Mukherjee et al. (1975).*

essential characteristics to be expected of the interaction of an
antagonist with the β-adrenergic receptors.   These include rapid
rates of association and dissociation of (-)[³H]dihydroalprenolol,
appropriate specificity, affinity, and saturability of (-)[³H]di-
hydroalprenolol binding (Mukherjee et al., 1975).

Figure 1 indicates the rapid forward and reverse rates of
binding of this ligand to erythrocyte membranes at 37°.   The kinetics of association are compatible with a simple bimolecular reaction.   From more extensive data than those shown in Figure 1, it
can be calculated that at 37° the forward rate constant for the bimolecular binding reaction is $k_1 = 1.84 \times 10^{-6} M^{-1} sec^{-1}$ and the reverse rate constant k_{-1} is $5.3 \times 10^{-3} sec^{-1}$.   Since $k_{-1}/k_1 = K_D$
(dissociation constant), it can be calculated from these kinetic
data that the dissociation constant of (-)[³H]dihydroalprenolol for
these binding sites is about 3 nM.   A comparable dissociation constant can be calculated from equilibrium studies of binding (Mukherjee et al., 1975; Mukherjee et al., 1976).

Figure 2 indicates that the binding of (-)[³H]dihydroalprenolol
to the membrane sites is a saturable process.   As noted, half-maximal occupancy of the sites occurs at about 3-5 nM (-)[³H]dihydro-

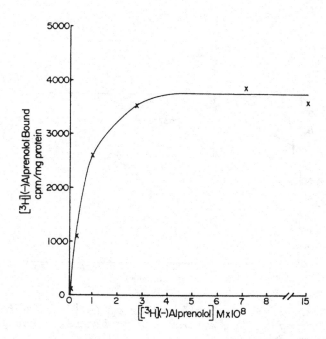

Figure 2. *(-)[³H]dihydroalprenolol binding to frog erythrocyte*
membranes is a function of increasing (-)[³H]dihydro-
alprenolol concentration. Taken from Mukerjee et al.,
1975.

alprenolol which corresponds to the K_D. The saturation-binding
value corresponds to about 1500 binding sites per intact frog
erythrocyte (Mukherjee *et al.*, 1975).

Specificity and affinity of $(-)[^3H]$dihydroalprenolol binding
as assessed by competition-binding experiments is quite comparable
to that for the interaction of antagonists with the adenylate
cyclase coupled to β-adrenergic receptors. Figure 3A demonstrates
the order of potency of the stereoisomers of β-adrenergic agonists
in stimulating the erythrocyte membrane adenylate cyclase. This
is (-)isoproterenol>(-)epinephrine>(-)norepinephrine. There is
also stereoselectivity in the response since the (+)isomer of each
of these agonists is considerable less effective than the (-)iso-
mer in activating the adenylate cyclase. Figure 3B demonstrates
the ability of each of these agents to compete for the $(-)[^3H]$di-
hydroalprenolol-binding sites. It is quite clear that this is
directly parallel to the dose-response curves for the stimulation
of adenylate cyclase by the β-adrenergic agonists. The same marked stereospecificity is also apparent. Comparable data were ob-

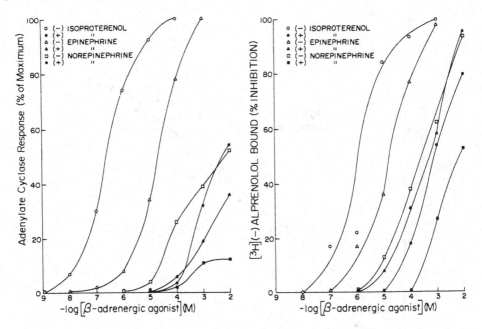

Figure 3. *A. Stimulation of frog erythrocyte membrane adenylate*
cyclase by β-adrenergic agonists. *B. Inhibition of*
(-)[³H]dihydroalprenolol binding to frog erythrocyte
membranes by β-adrenergic agonists. *From Mukherjee*
et al., 1975.

tained with β-adrenergic antagonists (Mukherjee *et al.*, 1975),
thus, the ability of a series of β-adrenergic antagonists to competitively inhibit isoproterenol-dependent adenylate cyclase
activity in these membranes directly parallels the ability of
these agents to compete for the (-)[³H]dihydroalprenolol binding
sites.

Using the frog erythrocyte membrane system we studied 60 β-adrenergic ligands with respect to their activation of the adenylate
cyclase system and their potency in competing with (-)[³H]dihydro-
alprenolol for the β-adrenergic binding sites (Mukherjee *et al.*,
1976). In all cases studied, the potency in the two assay systems
was directly parallel. Figure 4 is a plot of K_D values determined
in the binding assays versus the K_D determined in the adenylate
cyclase system. There is excellent agreement between the two sets
of data as indicated by the correlation coefficient of 0.95.

These data clearly indicate the essential equivalence of the

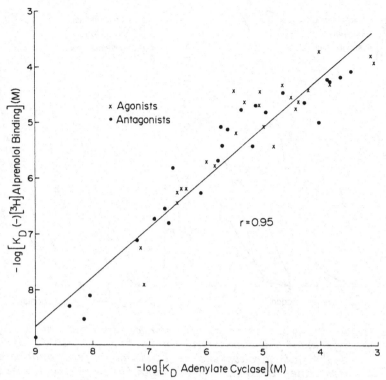

Figure 4. *Affinity constants of β-adrenergic agents for frog*
erythrocyte β-adrenergic receptors determined by direct
binding and adenylate cyclase studies. Taken from
Mukherjee et al., 1976.

properties of the $(-)[^3H]$dihydroalprenolol binding sites with the
characteristics expected of the physiological β-adrenergic receptors in the membranes. Comparable data have been obtained in a
wide variety of tissues including mammalian brain (Alexander *et
al.*, 1975), pineal gland (Zatz *et al.*, 1976), adipose tissue (Williams *et al.*, 1976, cardiac tissue (Alexander *et al.*, 1975), and
human lymphocytes (Williams *et al.*, 1976). Using these methods,
the characteristics of the β-adrenergic receptor binding sites
have been probed. The sites have been shown to exhibit negative
cooperativity (Limbird, De Meyts, and Lefkowitz, 1975) in some
systems such as the frog erythrocyte but not in others, such as
the turkey erythrocyte (Brown *et al.*, 1976), or mammalian brain
(Bylund and Snyder, 1976). In addition, the sites have been
characterized in biochemical terms, exhibiting lipoprotein properties (Limbird and Lefkowitz, 1976), and also these receptors have
been solubilized from the membranes (Caron and Lefkowitz, 1976).
These binding sites appear to reside in the plasma membranes of
adipose tissue cells and, therefore, $(-)[^3H]$dihydroalprenolol

prenolol binding may prove to be a very useful plasma membrane marker (Williams *et al.*, 1976).

Regulation of Adenylate Cyclase Coupled to β-Adrenergic Receptors

The ability to study directly the β-adrenergic receptors with radio-ligand binding techniques has opened new experimental approaches for the investigation of the physiological regulation of catecholamine responsiveness of tissues. It is a well known physiological observation that chronic exposure of tissues to high concentrations of certain hormones and drugs leads to tolerance or desensitization of the tissue to the biological effects of that particular agent. Such desensitization has been described with such diverse agents as opiates (Collier, 1966), insulin (Gavin, Roth, Neville, De Meyts, and Buell, 1974), cholinergic drugs (Miledi and Potter, 1971), and catecholamines (Remold-O'Donnell, 1974). Several groups have now reported that *in vitro* exposure of various cell types to catecholamines leads to decreased sensitivity of the membrane-bound adenylate cyclase to subsequent β-adrenergic stimulation (Franklin and Foster, 1973; Makman, 1971; Mickey, Tate, and Lefkowitz, 1975; Mukherjee, Caron, and Lefkowitz, 1975; Remold, 1974). Until recently, however, no information has been available concerning the molecular mechanisms involved in such desensitization. We have been studying this desensitization phenomenon in the frog erythrocyte model system. When frogs are injected with catecholamines (Mukherjee *et al.*, 1975) or when frog erythrocytes are incubated *in vitro* with catecholamines (Mickey *et al.*, 1975) there is a striking and selective fall in erythrocyte membrane adenylate cyclase responsiveness to subsequent stimulation by isoproterenol. Figure 5A demonstrates that this desensitization constitutes a decrease in the V_{max} of catecholamine-stimulated activity with no change in the apparent K_m for isoproterenol activation of this enzyme. Moreover, the desensitization is specific since there is no change in basal, fluoride-stimulated or prostaglandin E_1-sensitive enzyme activity (Figure 5B). Of further interest, prostaglandin E_1 desensitizes adenylate cyclase to subsequent prostaglandin stimulation without affecting catecholamine-sensitive enzyme activity. Figure 6A shows that when the β-adrenergic receptors in the desensitized membranes are studied directly with $(-)[^3H]$dihydroalprenolol a striking decrease in the apparent number of the sites was found with no alteration in the affinity (K_D) of the binding sites. In a large number of experiments the decrease in the number of sites was 68% after catecholamine treatment *in vivo* and 48% after treatment *in vitro* (Mickey *et al.*, 1975; Mukherjee *et al.*, 1975)(Figure 6B). Both of these values are statistically significant.

In order to gain insight into whether the catecholamine induced decrease in β-adrenergic receptors and in catecholamine-

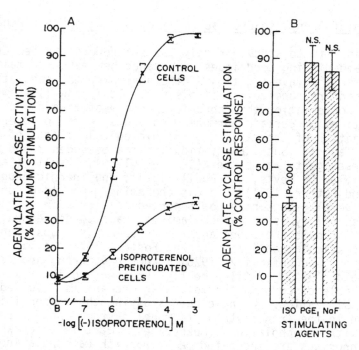

Figure 5A.   *Stimulation of frog erythrocyte membrane adenylate*
              cyclase by (-)isoproterenol in control cells and cells
              preincubated with isoproterenol. Adenylate cyclase as-
              says were performed with membranes derived from cells
              preincubated with or without (-)isoproterenol, 10^{-5} M,
              for five hours. Results shown are mean ± SEM from 10
              separate experiments. Taken from Mickey et al., 1975.

Figure 5B.   *Stimulation of frog erythrocyte membrane adenylate*
              cyclase from control and (-)isoproterenol-treated cells
              by (-)isoproterenol, prostaglandin E_1, and sodium flu-
              oride. Preincubations with (-)isoproterenol were per-
              formed as described in legend to Figure 5A. Concentra-
              tion of various stimulators in the assays were (-)iso-
              proterenol 10^{-4} M, prostaglandin E_1 10^{-5} M, and sodium
              fluoride 10 mM. NS = not statistically significant.
              Results shown are mean ± SEM from 10 experiments.
              Taken from Mickey et al., 1975.

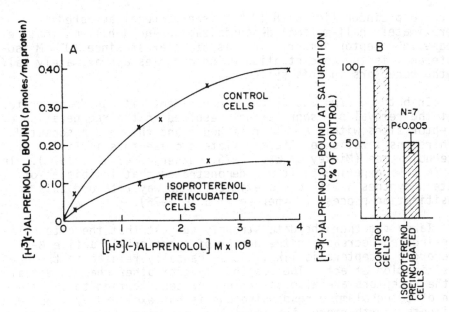

Figure 6A.   (-)[³H]dihydroalprenolol binding to membranes from
control and (-)isoproterenol-treated frog erythrocytes. Preincubation conditions were described in
Figure 5A.

Figure 6B.   Maximum (-)[³H]dihydroalprenolol binding to membranes
from control and (-)isoproterenol preincubated frog
erythrocytes. Binding was determined at high (8 x
10⁻⁸ M) (-)[³H]dihydroalprenolol concentrations.
Taken from Mickey et al., 1975.

sensitive adenylate cyclase activity were related, these two phenomena were further characterized in both *in vivo* (Mukherjee,
Caron, and Lefkowitz, 1976) and *in vitro* (Mickey, Tate, Mullikin,
and Lefkowitz, 1976) systems. It was found that in essentially
all characteristics studied the two effects were virtually identical. Thus, the specificity of the enzyme desensitization and
reduction in receptor binding sites were the same. Both were β-
adrenergic effects with isoproterenol causing the most desensitization and greatest decrease in receptor number. β-adrenergic
antagonists did not produce desensitization or a decrease in receptor number and, furthermore, the antagonists prevented the decrease in receptor number and desensitization seen after exposure
to β-adrenergic agonists. α-adrenergic antagonists did not act
in this manner. The time course of both phenomena was similar,
requiring about one hour for half-maximal desensitization *in vitro*.

In vitro preincubation with 10^{-6} M isoproterenol appeared to cause approximately half-maximal desensitization and a half-maximal decrease in receptor number. This is of interest since 10^{-6} M isoproterenol is the concentration which occupies approximately half of the receptors in this system.

In both *in vivo* and *in vitro* experiments it was demonstrated that the removal of isoproterenol resulted in the regeneration of receptor sites within a matter of hours and this was associated with resensitization of the adenylate cyclase to stimulation by catecholamines (Mickey *et al.*, 1976; Mukherjee *et al.*, 1976). In the *in vivo* experiments it was demonstrated that inhibition of protein synthesis with cycloheximide in no way retarded this resensitization process (Mukherjee *et al.*, 1976).

Taken together the data strongly suggest that the catecholamine-induced decrease in the number of functionally active β-adrenergic receptors is likely to be causally related to the desensitization effect. The possibility that other changes distal to the receptors are also occurring and contributing to the reduction of catecholamine-responsiveness is not excluded by these experiments. Furthermore, the molecular mechanisms by which β-adrenergic catecholamines cause these regulatory effects remain to be fully elucidated. However, the recent demonstration that desensitization can be produced in a cell-free system employing isolated membranes from frog erythrocytes suggests that induced conformational alterations may be involved. Thus, the ability to study the β-adrenergic receptors by direct binding techniques provides an entirely new approach to the study of the mechanisms of catecholamine desensitization. Such direct radioligand binding studies should have wide usefulness in probing the biochemical mechanisms involved in the regulation of hormone responsiveness of various tissues by hormones and drugs.

ACKNOWLEDGEMENT

This work was supported by HEW Grant #HL 16037 and a grant-in-aid from the American Heart Association with funds contributed, in part, by the North Carolina Heart Association. Dr. Lefkowitz is an Established Investigator of the American Heart Association.

REFERENCES

Alquist, R.P. (1948) A study of the adrenotropic receptors. *Amer. J. Physiol.* 153:586-600.
Alexander, R.W., Davis, J.N., and Lefkowitz, R.J. (1975) Direct identification and characterization of β-adrenergic receptors in rat brain. *Nature* 258:437-440.

Alexander, R.W., Williams, L.T., and Lefkowitz, R.J. (1975) Iden-
    tification of cardiac β-adrenergic receptors by (-)[³H]al-
    prenolol binding. *Proc. Nat'l. Acad. Sci.* 72:1564-1568.
Atlas, D., Steer, M.L., and Levitzki, A. (1974) Stereospecific
    binding of propranolol and catecholamines to the β-adren-
    ergic receptor. *Proc. Nat'l. Acad. Sci.* 71:4246-4248.
Aurbach, G.D., Fedak, S.A., Woodard, C.J., Palmer, J.S., Hauser,
    D., and Troxler, F. (1974) β-adrenergic receptor: Stereo-
    specific interaction of iodinated β-blocking agent with
    high affinity site. *Science* 186:1223-1224.
Brown, E.M., Rodbard, D., Fedak, S.A., Woodard, C.J., and Aurbach,
    G.D. (1976) β-adrenergic receptor interactions. Direct com-
    parison of receptor interaction and biological activity.
    J. Biol. Chem. 251:1239-1246.
Bylund, D. and Snyder, S. (1976) *Beta* adrenergic binding in mem-
    brane preparations from mammalian brain. *Mol. Pharm.* 12:
    568-580.
Caron, M.G. and Lefkowitz, R.J. (1976) Solubilization and char-
    acterization of the β-adrenergic receptor binding sites of
    frog erythrocytes. *J. Biol. Chem.* 251:2374-2384.
Collier, H.O.J. (1966) Tolerance, physical dependence and recep-
    tors. *Adv. in Drug Res.* 3:171-188.
Cuatrecasas, P., Tell, G.P.E., Sica, V., Parikh, I., and Chang,
    K.J. (1974) Noradrenaline binding and the search for cate-
    cholamine receptors. *Nature* 247:92-97.
Franklin, T.J. and Foster, S.J. (1973) Hormone-induced desensiti-
    zation of hormonal control of cyclic AMP levels in human
    diploid fibroblasts. *Nature New Biol.* 246:146-148.
Gavin, J.R. III, Roth, J., Neville, D.M. Jr., DeMeyts, P., and
    Buell, D.N. (1974) Insulin-dependent regulation of insulin
    receptor concentrations: A direct demonstration in cell cul-
    ture. *Proc. Nat'l. Acad. Sci.* 71:84-88.
Lefkowitz, R.J. (1975) Identification of adenylate cyclase-
    coupled *beta*-adrenergic receptors with radiolabeled *beta*-
    adrenergic antagonists. *Biochem. Pharm.* 24:1651-1658.
Lefkowitz, R.J. (1974) Stimulation of catecholamine-sensitive ad-
    enylate cyclase by 5'-quanylyl-imidodiphosphate. *J. Biol.
    Chem.* 249:6119-6124.
Lefkowitz, R.J. (1976) The β-adrenergic receptor. *Life Sci.* 18:
    461-472.
Lefkowitz, R.J., Limbird, L.E., Mikherjee, C., and Caron, M.G.
    (1976) The *beta* adrenergic receptor and adenylate cyclase.
    Biomem. Rev. 457:1-39
Lefkowitz, R.J., Mikherjee, C., Coverstone, M., and Caron, M.G.
    (1974) Stereospecific [³H](-)-alprenolol binding sites,β -
    adrenergic receptors and adenylate cyclase. *Biochem. Biophys.
    Res. Commun.* 60:703-709.
Levitzki, A., Atlas, D., and Steer, M.L. (1974) The binding char-
    acteristics and number of β-adrenergic receptors on the turkey
    erythrocyte. *Proc. Nat'l. Acad. Sci.* 71:2773-2776.

Limbird, L.E., DeMeyts, P., and Lefkowitz, R.J. (1975) β-adrenergic receptors: Evidence for negative cooperativity. *Biochem. Biophys. Res. Commu.* **64**:1160-1168.

Limbird, L.E. and Lefkowitz, R.J. (1976) Adenylate cyclase-
coupled *beta* adrenergic receptors: Effect of membrane lipid-
perturbing agents on receptor binding and enzyme stimulation
by catecholamines. *Mol. Pharm.* **12**:559-567.

Makman, M.H. (1971) Properties of adenylate cyclase of lymphoid
cells. *Proc. Nat'l. Acad. Sci.* **68**:885-889.

Mickey, J.V., Tate, R., and Lefkowitz, R.J. (1975) Subsensitivity
of adenylate cyclase and decreased β-adrenergic receptor
binding after chronic exposure to (-)-isoproterenol *in vitro.*
J. Biol. Chem. **250**:5727-5729.

Mickey, J.V., Tate, R., Millikan, D., and Lefkowitz, R.J. (1976)
Regulation of adenylate cyclase-coupled *beta* adrenergic receptor binding sites by *beta* adrenergic catecholamines *in
vitro.* *Mol. Pharm.* **12**:409-419.

Miledi, R. and Potter, L.T. (1971) Isolation of the cholinergic
receptor protein of *Torpedo* electric tissue. *Nature* **229**:554-
557.

Mukherjee, C., Caron, M.G., Coverstone, M., and Lefkowitz, R.J.
(1975) Identification of adenylate cyclase-coupled β-adrenergic receptors in frog erythrocytes with (-)[³H]alprenolol.
J. Biol. Chem. **250**:4869-4876.

Mukherjee, C., Caron, M.G., and Lefkowitz, R.J. (1976) Regulation
of adenylate cyclase coupled *beta*-adrenergic receptors by
beta-adrenergic catecholamines. *Endocrinology* **99**:347-357.

Mukherjee, C., Caron, M.G., and Lefkowitz, R.J. (1975) Catecholamine-induced subsensitivity of adenylate cyclase associated
with loss of β-adrenergic receptor binding sites. *Proc.
Nat'l. Acad. Sci.* **72**:1945-1949.

Mukherjee, C., Caron, M.G., Millikan, D., and Lefkowitz, R.J.
(1976) Structure-activity relationships of adenylate cyclase-
coupled *beta* adrenergic receptors: Determination by direct
binding studies. *Mol. Pharm.* **12**:16-31.

Remold-O'Donnell, E. (1974) Stimulation and desensitization of
macrophage adenylate cyclase by prostaglandins and catecholamines. *J. Biol. Chem.* **249**:3615-3621.

Robison, G.A., Butcher, R.W., and Sutherland, E.W. (1971) *Cyclic
AMP.* pp. 150-151, Academic Press, New York.

Rosen, O.M., Erlichman, J., and Rosen, S.M. (1970) The structure-
activity relationships of adrenergic compounds that act on
the adenyl cyclase of the frog erythrocyte. *Mol. Pharm.* **6**:
524-531.

Williams, L.T., Jarett, L., and Lefkowitz, R.J. (1976) Adipocyte
β-adrenergic receptors. Identification and subcellular
localization by (-)-[³H]dehydroalprenolol binding. *J. Biol.
Chem.* **251**:3096-3104.

Williams, L.T., Snyderman, R., and Lefkowitz, R.J. (1976) Identification of β-adrenergic receptors in human lymphocytes by

(-)[^{3}H]alprenolol binding. *J. Clin. Invest.* 57:149-155.
Zatz, M., Kebabian, J.W., Romero, J.A., Lefkowitz, R.J., and Axel-
    rod, J. (1976) Pineal *beta* adrenergic receptor: Correla-
    tion of binding of ^{3}H-1-alprenolol with stimulation of adeny-
    late cyclase. *J. Pharm. and Exp. Therap.* 196:714-722.

DISCUSSION FOLLOWING DR. LEFKOWITZ'S TALK

Dr. Freed
   It looks very much like you don't need the desensitization to get the resensitization, in the earlier slides the antagonists seemed to induce a supersensitization of some kind. I wonder if the absolute increase in the number of sites induced by antagonists is similar before and after desensitization.

Dr. Lefkowitz
   I think what you're asking me is: Does propranolol by itself supersensitize even if you don't bother to desensitize in the first place? That has been a real bag of worms, which we have had a lot of trouble with. Suffice it to say that, every time we have systematically tried to study the problem, we get a negative answer. Based on the data we have, I would have to say there's no real supersensitivity. Let me give you somebody else's data bearing on this question of sensitivity and supersensitivity. Julius Axelrod's lab has been using some of these methods which we've developed, to look at the sensitivity of the *beta* receptor in the pineal gland. That's a very fascinating and unique system, and I don't know how familiar you are with it, but this is a system in which there's a *beta* adrenergic receptor in the pineal, which is linked to adenylate cyclase and cyclic AMP accumulation. This in turn appears, among other things, to be involved in the induction of specific enzymes, which are involved in, I believe, serotonin synthesis. Isoproterenol has the ability to induce this enzyme or stimulate its activity through cyclic AMP and adenyl cyclase stimulation. Axelrod and his coworkers have shown that there is a diurnal variation in the sensitivity of the system to catecholamine stimulation. They cycle the animals through 12 hours light and 12 hours dark. When the lights are off, the system desensitizes to catecholamines. Catecholamines don't stimulate adenylate cyclase very well, similar to what we showed you here. You turn on the lights and very rapidly within an hour the cyclase becomes sensitive to catecholamine stimulation. They found that there's also a diurnal variation in the pineal norepinephrine content, which is directly what you would predict from the kind of data I've just shown you, that is, as the norepinephrine level went up, the system desensitized, and what we've shown you is that high levels of agonists desensitized, and that's just what happened. Very recently they've used these methods to look at receptor number, and get just what you would predict from these data. As the norepinephrine level rises, receptor level falls, and as it falls, catecholamine sensitivity level falls, and then as the receptor level comes back up catecholamine sensitivity comes back up.

Dr. Forte
     I gather from your comments, then, that smooth muscle has not
been an appropriate model for supersensitivity.

Dr. Lefkowitz
     We haven't used it, but that may have been a tactical error
thus far.

Dr. Forte
     I'm sure you're aware that the area of hormonal supersensi-
tivity has developed from the pharmacologic research dealing with
smooth muscle.

Dr. Lefkowitz
     This might be a good model system for us to look at.

Dr. Forte
     I have a comment to make before I open for more questions.
There is another peptide hormone that exerts this phenomenon of
subsensitivity, and that is parathyroid hormone. Your dose-response curves for activation of the erythrocyte adenylate cyclase
look very much like our dose-response curves for activation of
renal cortical adenylate cyclase by parathyroid hormone *in vitro*
or the results of our *in vivo* studies in terms of phosphaturic
responses and urinary cyclic AMP responses. These studies have
been done in the vitamin D-deficient rat. Vitamin D deficiency
induces a state of severe hypocalcemia in the rat. Hypocalcemia
leads to a secondary elevation of circulating parathyroid hormone
so these animals are exposed to high concentrations of parathyroid
hormone, and it may be that the results we are seeing are a result
of alteration in receptors, either in numbers or changes in properties. I think the easiest explanation is an alteration in numbers of receptors, but that has an infinite variety of subsets of
mechanisms associated with it, of course.

Dr. Lefkowitz
     Absolutely. I think your comment is very well taken, and I
would like to make it clear that I am in no sense trying to propose a general mechanism here for hormone desensitization. I can
think right off the top of my head of at least three or four
mechanisms for which there is reasonable data in the literature
already which are different than this. I must say that our data
in some respects are very similar to what's been published with
certain of the polypeptide hormones like insulin. The major difference between our data and say, the insulin data is that there,
protein synthesis inhibition appears to have very marked effects,
that is to say, protein synthesis in addition markedly retards the
rate of regeneration of the receptors once you take isoproterenol
out of the system. In our system we can't really demonstrate that

frog erythrocytes make any protein. But granted that even in the
presence of protein synthesis inhibitors like cycloheximide the
regeneration of receptors occurs at the same rate. Thus, I sus-
pect, in our system, that the receptor inactivation, whatever the
mechanism, does not involve a true loss of the receptors from the
cell membranes. They don't have to be resynthesized; at least
that's our thinking.

Dr. Forte
     Does Dr. Burns have any comments about *alpha* receptors?

Dr. Burns
     No, but I would like to ask the speaker about the possibility
of solubilizing a receptor that would respond to catecholamines. I
know that two or three people around the country have reported doing this. You touched on it briefly, and I wonder if you'd just
say a little more about (a) the published results in which it is
claimed to have been done and (b) what you think the prognosis is
for these results to be confirmed elsewhere.

Dr. Lefkowitz
     I'm not sure that I understand specifically the question.
Are you referring to the reports of solubilization followed by
reconstitution with lipids?

Dr. Burns
     That's the one, and then I think Storm and Ryan reported
solubilization without reconstitution.

Dr. Lefkowitz
     Right, I'll comment on both of those results. It was report-
ed by Levey, starting in 1970, that adenylate cyclases could be
solubilized with Lubrol-PX, a specific detergent, and I think that
has been widely confirmed. He also reported that in his hands the
Lubrol-PX detergent-solubilized cyclases lost hormone sensitivity
in general when they were in the solubilized state and I think
that's been widely confirmed. What he then reported was that if
he removed the detergent by ion exchange chromatography and added
back specific phospholipids, he could then restore hormone sensitivity to the cyclase. He reported that phosphatidyl serine restored glucagon and histamine sensitivity and that monophosphatide
inositol specifically restored catecholamine stimulation. I think
it's fair to say that those data are not reproducible. We tried
for quite some time to reproduce them. There are in the literature several examples of "reconstituted cyclases," but in general
those have not involved solubilization. We found, for example,
that we could treat cardiac membranes with phospholipases and retain catalytic activity while losing hormone sensitivity. There
are similar reports in liver membranes, that have been published
as well. I accept the concept that lipids, at least in the sense

of the lipid matrix of the membranes, are crucially involved in
the coupling of hormone binding to cyclase. I am, however, very
reticent to accept the concept that there is the great specificity
that Levey implied, namely, this lipid gives you this hormone response, etc. It may or may not be true, but at least to me the
data available thus far are more consistent with the notion that
lipids play a more general role, perhaps in maintaining a membrane
environment or something like this. In terms of the report of
Storm and Ryan in BBRC, we haven't tried to reproduce their finding. However, based on our findings and the findings of one or
two other investigators that I'm aware of, I don't think there
will be anything magical about that detergent, that is, the detergent (Triton X-305) is not going to prove to be the magic bullet
that solubilizes hormone-sensitive adenylate cyclases.

Dr. Forte
     I might speak to that. We did try to solubilize with that
detergent, Triton X-305, and found that the detergent was a poor
solubilizing agent for membrane proteins. At the concentrations
of the detergent that were used, we found a minimal inhibitory
action of the detergent on hormone responsiveness. However, if
you truly separate a soluble membrane protein fraction, then that
protein fraction will exhibit fluoride-stimulated but not hormone-
dependent adenylate cyclase activity. So I think that Triton
X-305 produces the same dissociation of hormone-responsiveness
while maintaining fluoride-activation of the adenylate cyclase
that has been with other Tritons, Lubrol, and sodium deoxycholate.

Dr. Hechter
     One comment, and then a question. The data that you've re-
ported on desensitization and recovery of receptor function is
very reminiscent of findings in pharmacology that are subsumed
under the title of tachyphylaxis. Anyone who has worked with
uterotonic assays to measure the activity of a contractile agent
(be it oxytocin, prostaglandins, angiotensin, bradykinin), learns
that there are certain "rules" one must follow to get reproducible
dose response curves. Thus, after an agonist is added in high
concentration and contraction has been evoked, the agonist is then
rapidly "washed out" of the bath; if you do not do this, and the
agonist acts for 5 or 10 minutes, the uterine dose-response relationship may become chaotic. The tissue can exhibit hypersensi-
tivity to previously ineffective doses; alternatively the tissue
may become nonresponsive to the specific agonist, so that doses
previously effective are now ineffective (tachyphylaxis). Workers
experienced in the uterotonic assay, have long felt that there
might well be low affinity "storage sites" in the uterus which
bind agonists, but are not directly related to the receptors involved in hormone (or agonist) action. If there be such "storage
sites" in the neighborhood of receptor sites, it is possible that
occupation of these storage sites, may lead to modification of re-

ceptor sites via one mechanism or another. The possibility arises
that the low affinity "nonspecific" binding sites generally detected in membranes with radioactive hormone ligands correspond,
in part, to these "storage sites."

Now the question: You can measure specific binding to β-
adrenergic receptors in frog membranes and a variety of other
catecholamine-responsive membranes; you can also measure adenylate cyclase activation. Have you studied the kinetics of enzyme
activation in relation to the kinetics of occupation under identical incubation conditions? I think you mentioned that in the
frog membrane there is a linear relationship between hormone occupation and enzyme activation. Is this true for other systems
such as the fat cell membrane?

Dr. Lefkowitz
     It's true for the frog membrane, and I don't know if it's
true for any other membrane because we've not done the kind of
detailed kinetic analysis that you described for any other system.
Let me make two comments in response to Dr. Hechter's remarks.
One is that in terms of tachyphylaxis I think it's important, and
I think we're speaking about the same thing, that there are all
different kinds of desensitization mechanisms. There's what's
been called fatigue-type phenomena, there is toxicity--if you put
a high enough concentration of anything on anything the system
dies, that's no big wonder. The key to what we're talking about
is a very specific desensitization. I have no experience with
these uterotonic assays you're talking about, but the analogy in
such a system would be that, let's say there were four different
agonists, different types of agonists that stimulated it. To
fulfill the kind of phenomena that I think I'm talking about it
would have to be a phenomenon where, let's say, you put oxytocin
on there and now you either wash or you don't wash, and look, it
doesn't respond so well to oxytocin. Now you take methylcholine,
you put that on, beautiful response. It's got to be a desensitization which is hormone-specific. In other words, at a time when
this system is desensitized to catecholamines, basal, fluoride,
prostaglandin-stimulated activities, they're perfect, so I think
there are analogies in that respect. There is a totally different
phenomenon described by Ho and Sutherland in fat cells where, if
you stimulate with epinephrine and then try to rechallenge at a
certain period of time later, you can't challenge with epinephrine
or glucagon. There seems to be production of what they call a
feedback inhibitor. We're not talking about that kind of mechanism
because that's not specific, and that seems to me unlikely to involve the receptors.

     The thing about the curved Scatchard plots is a very compli-
cated issue that I think it would be difficult to go into at this
time. There are some hormone receptors for which Scatchard plots

are straight. For example, growth hormone binding to its receptors appears to give a straight Scatchard plot. The kind of
binding I've shown you in several of our other systems is not
curved the way it is here, but as Dr. Hechter says, one reason
for curved Scatchard plots is more than one order of site where
one order of site might be the receptor, one order of site might
be something else. Both orders of site might be the receptors,
or there might even be many orders of sites. Another reason for
curved Scatchard plots, which has been clearly shown now is cooperative interactions between the sites. For example, we have
independent evidence from several different lines that there are
negatively cooperative interactions among these *beta* adrenergic
receptors in frog erythrocytes. I'll give you a layman's defini-
tion of cooperativity. From a layman's point-of-view, the oppo-
site of cooperative interactions would be all the sites are independent, that is, the filling of any one or number of the sites by
ligands in no way influences the statistical likelihood or probability that the other sites will become filled at any given concentration of hormone. The sites are independent. In a cooperative system this isn't so. In a cooperative system there are interactions among the sites such that as you fill the sites the
empty sites change their affinity. In a negatively cooperative
system it would mean that as you fill the sites, the sites which
are still empty become less likely to bind because of negatively
cooperative interactions. In a Scatchard plot you would see just
what you saw here, namely that as you got down toward the bottom
of the plot, as the sites are now largely filled, the remaining
empty sites have a lowered affinity. From Scatchard plots alone
you cannot distinguish those, and I wouldn't attempt to. We have
independent kinetic evidence that there is negative cooperativity
here, which have to do with the dissociation rates of the label
from the sites in the presence and absence of a large excess of
unlabelled ligand, but I won't go into that unless there is somebody who particularly wants me to.

Dr. Klachko

I heard some suggestions in Dr. Lefkowitz's talk that Dr.
Hechter's suggested storage sites might, in fact, be in the re-
ceptor-activated complex. In other words, although all these
agonists and antagonists will bind because of the common sidechain,
apparently only a random third will switch on the system. The rest
of the molecule probably is important, then, for a conformational
change, which either may be complete or partial and leading to
partial activation of the enzyme. Perhaps that agonist is then
trapped in that conformational change and requires relaxation and
release before the system can be reactivated. Even though Dr.
Lefkowitz said that it was impossible to wash off the isoproterenol, I wonder if he has perhaps looked at labelled isoproterenol
and seen whether it is still trapped there and whether the release
can be facilitated by an antagonist with reconstitution of the

sensitivity of the system.

Dr. Lefkowitz
We can only get at parts of that question. I've avoided say-
ing anything about the molecular mechanism of this receptor inactivation. One possibility would be that agonists, when they bind
to the receptor, in some way become trapped in some sort of tight
complex with the receptor, which is clearly not easily reversible,
and at the same time the complex is also not active. I'm not
quite sure how to get at that. We deliberately avoided doing the
labelled isoproterenol experiment because I don't like to do experiments that I can't interpret. It's been amply demonstrated
that labelled isoproterenol binds to all kinds of sites, receptors and others, the function and nature of which are largely,
at this time, unspecified and unknown. So if I put the labelled
isoproterenol on, washed extensively, and found a few counts or
some counts, I just wouldn't know what to make of it because I
wouldn't know where they were bound. I don't think the mechanism
of receptor inactivation is some sort of chronic occupancy. It's
a possibility, though. All we can say is that the sites are inactivated. Whether they're inactivated because they're quasi-ir-
reversibly occupied we can't say.

Dr. DeGroot
Is there a phenomenon like capping with your receptors? Do
you know whether there's any mobility of the receptors?

Dr. Lefkowitz
We just have no data on that point. We wondered about it ourselves, but we just haven't approached it experimentally.

Dr. DeGroot
If you remove your catechol from the system, if you dilute it,
you get very rapid release of the catechol, right?

Dr. Lefkowitz
Yes, that's right.

Dr. DeGroot
Is the downslope of the adenylcyclase activity the same as
that?

Dr. Lefkowitz
I don't have good quantitative data on that, so I can't say.

Dr. DeGroot
Does the adenylcyclase stimulation depend entirely on the
presence of the catecholamine or is it stimulated for a longer period of time?

Dr. Lefkowitz
     Yes, it does depend continuously for the activated state on
the presence of the isoproterenol. For example, let's say you
have a certain basal cyclase rate. Cyclic AMP is gradually being
generated. Now you add isoproterenol. Within a minute the slope
is going up at a very steep rate. Now add propranolol. Within
30 seconds you've resumed basal rate. In other words, as soon as
the isoproterenol is removed from the receptor, that's it, you're
back to basal, so the activated state continuously requires the
presence of isoproterenol on the receptor.

Dr. DeGroot
     The third question is a little more complicated. I take it
with your desensitization experiments you have continuous exposure.
First, you put in lots of your agonist and you get a hyperactive
state. Now if you continue the exposure in that activation, then
both the adenylcyclase and receptor activity goes down, is that
right? Now you wash it out and you cannot find all of the original receptors.

Dr. Lefkowitz
     And you cannot find the amount of catecholamine stimulation
that you were previously able to get.

Dr. DeGroot
     Right. You find only some of the receptors left. My question
is, are their kinetic characteristics and binding characteristics
and affinity the same as the ones that were there, are they like a
part of the ones that were there originally, or are they different
afterwards?

Dr. Lefkowitz
     I feel confident that I can answer that question by saying
yes, their characteristics are identical. There are just less of
them, and we've looked at that in detail in a variety of different
ways with kinetic and equilibrium studies. The characteristics of
the sites that are left are identical to what we started with, it's
just that there are 50% or less of them there.

Dr. Kornel
     Among the other possibilities, could desensitization phenomena
be the result of an exhaustion of one or more cofactors?

Dr. Lefkowitz
     Well, we're always getting into semantics. If it's exhaustion,
I mean, it's a matter of how do we conceive of the system. Well,
we conceive of the system as being an enzyme complex, a membrane-
bound enzyme complex to adenylate cyclase, and we also conceive of
the system as containing receptors or discriminators or whatever
you want to call them. Some say there must be other parts to the

system, "couplers." If there's exhaustion, it's not exhaustion of the enzyme because the enzyme's fine. It's certainly not exhaustion of general type couplers in the sense that other hormones stimulate just fine; other hormones have to be coupled in too. So if there is exhaustion, it's exhaustion either of the receptors or the couplers or, as you would call it, some cofactor involved in receptors or coupling.

Dr. Kornel
      You haven't examined this yet?

Dr. Lefkowitz
      No, largely because one doesn't know exactly what the nature of any such cofactors are.

Dr. Hechter
      You had one slide that was intriguing. You had a partial agonist, which gave some fraction of maximal adenylate cyclase activity. However, when you study competitive binding against your radioactive ligand, that partial agonist completely inhibited occupation.

Dr. Lefkowitz
      Right.

Dr. Hechter
      Now you said this means the partial agonist occupies all the sites.

Dr. Lefkowitz
      Right.

Dr. Hechter
      I think that two possibilities must be considered: the partial agonist may occupy all sites as you suggest; alternatively, the agent could prevent the ligand from occupying these sites by another mechanism, without the partial agonist occupying all receptor sites. How does one explain the activity of a partial agonist which occupies all receptor sites, when you have shown us an elegant linear relationship between specific binding and adenylate cyclase activation?

Dr. Lefkowitz
      I can't answer that question. It basically gets down to the question of once you occupy a receptor, how do you turn the system on? For example, let's take propranolol or an antagonist; it occupies all the receptors and it doesn't turn anything on. Then there's isoproterenol, which occupies all the receptors, and turns everything on. And then there are these other compounds you're talking about, which occupy all the receptors and only turn it on a

little, and that's to me the biggest unknown in the whole thing.
It may depend on how much of a conformational change the agent can
cause. Isoproterenol turns all the receptors into some conforma-
tionally different state which then activates the cyclase. Propranolol occupies them all and you know doesn't turn them all on,
and then this one causes an intermediate amount. All the partial
agonists, as you would predict from classical pharmacological
theory, and as we can ourselves document, are also antagonists.
When you put in one of these partial agonists and it doesn't stimulate further, it will block isoproterenol at that point because
it's on the receptors, and you can show that it's there and occupy-
ing all the receptors by the fact that it will then block isoproterenol. The correlation that we have between the ability of partial agonists to only partially stimulate the cyclase and only
partially desensitize intrigues me, but I can't quite get a handle
on it. In other words, it says to me that just as agonism is a
measure of the ability to cause a conformational change or generate a message, so too desensitization is a function of some message or signal generated at the receptor, which antagonists can't
do because they're just antagonists. I think that the message, if
there is such a message, is not anything as simple as "well, it's
just cyclic AMP." Prostaglandin leads to cyclic AMP accumulation,
but that doesn't desensitize the *beta* receptor. Well, then maybe
you could say that you need cyclic AMP generated and the receptor
occupied, maybe that's it. At the moment our current thinking is
we're trying to see if we can study this in a cell-free system,
and it appears that we can. We can reproduce this phenomenon in a
cell-free system in just membranes. Maybe we'll be able to progress further in terms of mechanism there.

STUDIES OF ACETYLCHOLINE RECEPTOR PROTEIN

Robert N. Brady and William M. Moore

Department of Biochemistry
Vanderbilt University
Nashville, TN 37232

INTRODUCTION

The transfer of excitation from nerve to muscle fibers is one of the most thoroughly studied examples of chemical transmission in the nervous system. A great deal is now known about the storage, release, and metabolism of acetylcholine, the neurotransmitter involved in the transmission of impulses at the neuromuscular junction. However, there is still inadequate information about the nature of the acetylcholine binding sites of the postsynaptic membrane, how they are integrated into the cell membranes, and how the events initiated at these receptors may be coupled to ionic, electrical potential, biochemical and mechanical changes.

It is now well established that the response of an excitable membrane to acetylcholine and to cholinergic agonists involves a selective increase of permeability to cations (Katz, 1966) which is blocked by a class of related compounds, the cholinergic antagonists. Acetylcholine acts, therefore, as a regulatory ligand controlling membrane permeability.

The concept that soluble, regulatory proteins often exist as multiple-subunit allosteric enzymes is important to understanding the action of acetylcholine. These enzymes achieve their effects by the conformational changes that occur when a specific ligand small-molecule binds to one of the subunits. Similarly, subunit-containing proteins embedded in a membrane could provide a plausible mechanism for many important membrane phenomena that are not adequately understood at present. As is the case with nerve impulse transmission, any of these phenomena involve a change in a membrane function or property that accompanies the binding of some

apparently unrelated molecule. It has been postulated that the
action of acetylcholine is mediated by a minimum of two distinct
structural elements: a "receptor" protein which recognizes cholinergic agonists and an "ionophore" which accounts for the selective translocation of ions, and which could be either a region
of the receptor protein or a distinct, but tightly coupled, entity
(Changeux, Blumenthal, Kasai, and Podleski, 1970). In this hypothesis, a conformational transition (Nachmansohn, 1959) would control the interaction between the acetylcholine receptor and ionophore components. The elucidation of this cholinergic mechanism
awaits the complete identification and characterization of the components involved. Such studies are currently underway in many laboratories throughout the world (for review see deRobertis and
Schacht, 1974; Rang, 1973).

The acetylcholine receptors of skeletal muscles were called
"nicotinic" by Dale because they could be distinguished from other
cholinergic-binding sites by pharmacological means. They (like
those of electric tissues) are activated by nicotine and antagonized
competitively by d-tubocurarine. A direct approach to the selective
isolation and purification of these nicotinic receptors requires the
use of specific affinity ligands. Elapid snake venoms contain polypeptide neurotoxins which possess the extraordinary properties of
binding with very high affinity and with nearly total specificity to
the nicotinic acetylcholine receptor (AChR)[1] found in excitable membranes at neuromuscular junctions (Boquet, Izard, Jouannet, and
Meaume, 1966; Lee and Chang, 1966). For most studies of the fine
structural organization of receptors in muscles, α-bungarotoxin
from the krait *Bungarus multicinctus* has proved most satisfactory.
For other purposes, such as the assay for the purification of AChR
after its solubilization from membrane preparations, the more reversible α-toxins from cobra have been employed with equal success.
These α-toxins are small (MW 6700-7800), stable, basic polypeptides,
representing 10%-40% of the protein of the venom. They are readily
purified and retain biological activity when chemically modified by
the introduction of an isotopic label. Therefore, the alliance of
two war-like creatures, elapid snakes and electric fish (a rich
source of AChR), has led to the rather rapid accumulation of new
knowledge concerning cholinergic transmission.

Materials and Methods

Lyophilized venoms of *Naja naja atra* (Formosan cobra), *Naja
naja siamensis* (Thailand cobra), and *Bungarus multicinctus* (Formo-

---

[1]Abbreviations used are: AChR, acetylcholine receptor; OV,
ovalbumin; Ald, aldolase, Chym, chymotrypsinogen; RNase A, ribo-
nuclease A.

san krait) were supplied by the Ross Allen Reptile Institute, Silver Springs, Florida. Cyanogen bromide activated Sepharose 4B, SP-Sephadex, DEAE Sephadex, and Sephadex G-100 were purchased from Pharmacia, Uppsala, Sweden. *Torpedo nobiliana* was obtained from the Marine Biological Laboratory, Woods Hole, Massachusetts.

Protein was determined by amino acid analysis on a Beckman Model 121 amino acid analyzer according to the procedure of Shih and Hash (1971), and by the method of Lowry, Rosebrough, Farr, and Randall (1951). Acetylcholinesterase activity was determined by measuring the rate of acetylthiocholine hydrolysis as described by Ellman, Courtney, Andres, and Featherstone (1961). Amino-acid analysis was carried out on a Beckman Model 121 amino-acid analyzer with a norleucine internal standard (Liu and Chang, 1971). Absorption and circular dichroism spectra were obtained with an Hitachi-Perkin-Elmer EPS-3T spectrophotometer and a Cary 60 spectropolarimeter with a circular dichroism attachment, respectively.

Preparation of Electroplax and Particulate Fractions. Electric organs were excised from freshly killed *Torpedo nobiliana* and homogenized for 0.5 minutes in a Waring blender. The homogenate was lyophilized and stored at -70°C. No loss of receptor activity was observed after prolonged storage of material processed in this manner.

Particulate fractions from *T. nobiliana* were prepared in the following manner. Lyophilized electric organ tissue (250 mg) was suspended in 10 ml of modified Ringer's solution (Karlin, 1967), and homogenized in a Ten Broeck hand homogenizer. The resulting suspension was centrifuged for one hour at 36,000 x g and the pellet retained. Brain particulate fractions were obtained by decapitating male Sprague Dawley rats (180-220 grams) and homogenizing whole brains in ice cold 0.32 M sucrose, 0.001 M EDTA, 0.05 M sodium phosphate, pH 7.4 (10 ml/g brain). The homogenate was centrifuged at 34,800 x g for 20 minutes at 0°. The resulting pellet was either resuspended in 0.05 M sodium phosphate, pH 7.4, at 23° and used for subsequent studies of particulate-bound receptor or used directly to prepare soluble AChR preparations (see below).

Extraction of Particulate Fractions. Receptor protein was extracted from *T. nobiliana* membranes by stirring the membrane suspension with 1% Triton X-100 in Ringer's solution (v/v) at room temperature for one hour, followed by centrifugation for one hour at 36,000 x g. The resulting supernatant solution routinely contained 80% of the neurotoxin-binding activity originally present in the excitable membranes. The rat brain particulate pellet was (1) resuspended in 10 volumes of 0.05 M sodium phosphate buffer, pH 7.4; (2) recentrifuged at 34,800 x g for 20 minutes at 0°; (3) stirred for two hours at 23° with 1% Emulphogene BC-720, 0.05 M

sodium phosphate buffer, pH 7.4; and (4) recentrifuged at 34,800
x g for 20 minutes. Approximately 80%-90% of the rat brain AChR
activity was solubilized by this procedure.

Preparation of Neurotoxins. The principal neurotoxins of
B. *multicinctus* (α-bungarotoxin) and *N.n. siamensis* were prepared
as reported by Ong and Brady (1974). Cobratoxin was isolated from
the venom of *N.n. atra* according to Yang (1964). Each neurotoxin
was shown to be homogeneous by disc gel electrophoresis (Reisfeld,
Lewis, and Williams, 1962).

Radioactive α-toxins. Tritium was incorporated into the α-
toxins of *N.n. siamensis* and *N.n. atra* (cobra toxin) by reductive
formylation (Rice and Means, 1971) utilizing ^{3}H-sodium borohydride
as the reducing agent. Incorporation of ^{125}I into α-bungarotoxin
was achieved by lactoperoxidase catalyzed iodination (Morrison and
Bayse, 1970). Disc gel electrophoresis (Reisfeld *et al.*, 1962) of
the purified radioactive α-toxins displayed single bands which ran
concurrently with native toxin. All radioactivity corresponded in
position to the visible protein band. Precipitation (see Methods)
of ^{3}H-toxin-receptor complex in the presence of excess solubilized
T. nobiliana receptor revealed that 70% of the toxin molecules retained AChR-binding ability. Similar studies utilizing the DE-81
anion exchange filter disc assay (see Methods) demonstrated that
75% of the labeled ^{125}I-α-bungarotoxin molecules retained the ability to bind soluble *T. nobiliana* AChR. The neurotoxic properties
of the ^{3}H-α-toxins as judged by time to complete blockade in the
rat phrenic nerve diaphragm preparation (Bilbring, 1946) were reduced to 75% of those of the native toxin. The specific radioactivity was 1.9 Ci/mmole for ^{3}H-cobratoxin and 8.1 Ci/mmole for the
α-toxin of *N.n. siamensis*. The specific radioactivity of ^{125}I-α-
bungarotoxin was determined to be 32 Ci/mmole.

Preparation of Selective Adsorbents. Neurotoxins were coupled
to cyanogen bromide activated Sepharose 4B essentially according to
Axen, Porath, and Ernbach (1967) as modified by Ong and Brady
(1974). The coupling reaction was determined to be 92% complete
and approximately 10% of the coupled toxin residues retained the
ability to bind soluble AChR protein.

Assay for Toxin-AChR Complex. The extent of complex formation
of ^{3}H-toxin or ^{125}I-toxin with soluble *T. nobiliana* AChR was assayed either by a modification of the ammonium sulfate precipitation
method of Franklin and Potter (1972) or by the DE-81 anion exchange
filter disc method of Schmidt and Raftery (1973). Soluble brain
^{125}I-toxin-AChR complex formation was determined by shaking at 23°
aliquots of soluble brain extract with 1% Emulphogene, 0.05 M sodium phosphate, pH 7.4, and 12.6 x 10^{-9} M ^{125}I-toxin (2ml volume).
At the end of one hour 8 ml of 37.5% saturated ammonium sulfate was
added to each sample, mixed well, and the resulting precipitate

was immediately collected by filtration through Whatman F-G/B
glass fiber filter circles. The precipitate was washed with 15
ml of 30% saturated ammonium sulfate and radioactivity determined by counting the filter discs in a γ-ray spectrometer.

Binding of ^{125}I-α-bungarotoxin to particulate fractions of
rat brain was determined by shaking aliquots of the particulate
fraction (see Preparation of Electroplax and Particulate Fraction) with ^{125}I-α-bungarotoxin for one hour at 23°. Controls were
carried out by treating samples under identical incubation conditions with native α-bungarotoxin, prior to the addition of ^{125}I-
toxin. Incubation with ^{125}I-α-bungarotoxin was terminated by centrifugation at 34,800 x g for 20 minutes at 0°C. Supernatants
were discarded and pellets washed twice by resuspension in 10 ml
of 0.05 M sodium phosphate, pH 7.4. Washed pellets were then resuspended in 5 ml of 0.05 M sodium phosphate and aliquots counted
in a Nuclear Chicago γ-ray spectrometer.

Affinity Chromatography. Affinity columns (0.5 x 4.5 cm)
were prepared in glass wool-stoppered Pasteur pipets. To insure
maximal adsorption of the AChR, solubilized AChR preparations were
cycled through the column twice. The column was then washed with
the following series of eluents: 3.0 ml modified Ringer's; 3.0
ml of 1.0 M sodium chloride in 0.05 M potassium phosphate buffer,
pH 7.0; and 3.0 ml 0.05 M potassium phosphate buffer, pH 7.0. Each
wash solution contained 1% Triton X-100.

The affinity column was connected in series to a Pasteur
pipet column (0.5 x 4.5 cm) of DEAE-Sephadex A-25. A solution of
0.1 M carbamylcholine chloride in 0.01 M potassium phosphate buffer, pH 7.0, and 1% Triton X-100 was then cycled from a reservoir,
through the columns and returned to the reservoir by means of a
Technicon pump (flow rate, 0.25 ml/minute; see Figure 1). During
elution the temperature was maintained at 4°. The DEAE-Sephadex
column was removed from the system after specified time periods
(one, two, or three days) and was washed with 5.0 ml of 0.01 M
potassium phosphate buffer, pH 7.0, 0.1% Triton X-100 to completely remove the cycling eluent. The purified AChR was displaced
from the DEAE-Sephadex with 0.5 M sodium chloride in 0.01 M potassium phosphate buffer, pH 7.0, 0.1% Triton X-100. Fractions of
1.0 ml were collected; 70%-80% of the recovered AChR was obtained
in the first ml of the column eluate.

Polyacrylamide Gel Electrophoresis. SDS gel electrophoresis
was performed according to the procedure of Weber and Osborn
(1969). Molecular weights were established by coelectrophoresis
with standards. Densitometric traces were obtained using a Gil-
ford spectrophotometer with a Model 2410 linear transport attachment.

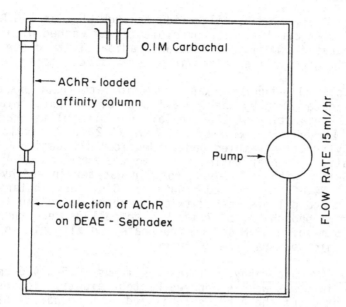

Figure 1.   Continuous elution affinity chromatography (see Methods).

RESULTS--ELECTRIC TISSUE

Formation of ³H-cobratoxin-AChR Complex. The elution profile
obtained by chromatography of solubilized ³H-cobratoxin-AChR complex (see Legend, Figure 2) on Sephadex G-100 is shown in Figure 2.
A clean separation of ³H-cobratoxin-AChR complex from ³H-cobratoxin
is achieved by this procedure. An identical pattern is obtained if
the ³H-cobratoxin is added to the extract after the excitable membranes have been solubilized. As indicated in Figure 3, formation
of the ³H-cobratoxin-AChR complex is linear with respect to added
solubilized membrane protein over the concentration range examined.
The extent of complex formation is greatly decreased when either
d-tubocurare, carbachol, or the neurotoxin of *N.n. siamensis* are
included in the assay mixture. As seen in Table 1, saturated concentrations of d-tubocurare (10^{-2} M) only reduce complex formation
by 62% whereas high levels of carbachol and *N.n. siamensis* neurotoxin essentially abolish ³H-cobratoxin-AChR complex formation.
Of the latter two ligands, the neurotoxin is by far the more potent, completely inhibiting complex formation when added at a concentration 20 times that of the ³H-cobratoxin. High salt and
lysozyme, a protein of low molecular weight and high pI, have no
measurable effect on complex formation.

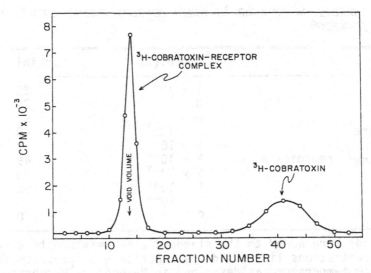

Figure 2. *Chromatography of solubilized membrane protein on Sep-*
hadex G-100. A preparation of crude Torpedo *electro-*
plax membranes was maximally labeled with [³H] cobra-
toxin, then washed extensively by centrifugation to re-
move free toxin. The membranes were extracted with
Triton X-100 as described in Methods and the solubil-
ized protein obtained after centrifugation was submit-
ted to gel chromatography. Fractions of 5.0 ml were
collected and radioactivity determined. [Reprinted
with permission from D.E. Ong and R.N. Brady (1974)
Biochem. *13:2822. Copyright by the American Chemical*
Society.]

Reversal of ³H-cobratoxin-AChR Complex. The ability of
various neuroactive agents to reverse the H-cobratoxin-AChR complex is summarized in Table 2. Carbachol, decamethonium, and d-
tubocurare very efficiently displace the toxin from the complex.
Since the extent of complex reversal is not linear with respect to
the concentration of displacing agent, no direct comparisons can
be made concerning the relative efficiencies of these three ligands
to displace cobratoxin from the complex. The neurotoxins of *N.n.*
siamensis and *B. multicinctus* effectively reversed the complex when
added at a concentration 100 times that of the ³H-cobratoxin. High
salt and lysozyme (at concentration 200 times that of the cobratoxin) have no measurable effect on complex reversal.

When the complex was partially reversed with carbachol and the
assay mixture was applied directly to a column of DEAE Sephadex A-25,

Table 1.   *INHIBITION OF AChR-³H-TOXIN COMPLEX FORMATION BY VARIOUS*
            LIGANDS[a]

Ligand	Concn.(M)	Inhibition(%)
Carbachol	1×10^{-4}	25
	0.1	78
	0.5	97
d-Tubocurare	1×10^{-3}	49
	1×10^{-2}	62
N.n. siamensis neurotoxin	1×10^{-8}	49
	5×10^{-7}	83
	1×10^{-5}	96
Lysozyme	1×10^{-4}	0
NaCl	0.5	0

[a]Ligands were added to the standard assay mixture to give the ligand concentrations listed and the reaction was incubated for one hour at room temperature as described in Methods. ³H-cobratoxin was added (5×10^{-7} M) and the reaction was incubated for an additional hour. The final volume was 2.0 ml. The per cent inhibition was determined by the decrease in precipitate counts compared to the assay without added ligand. [Reprinted with permission from D.E. Ong and P.N. Brady (1974) *Biochem.* 13:2822. Copyright by the American Chemical Society.]

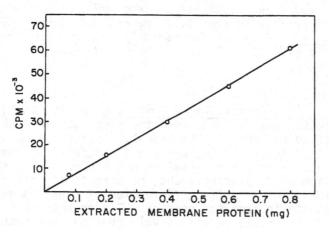

Figure 3.   *Formation of ³H-toxin-AChR complex. Increasing amounts of extracted membrane protein were added to 3.0 x 10⁻⁷ M ³H-cobratoxin and assayed for complex formation as described in Methods. [Reprinted with permission from D.E. Ong and R.N. Brady (1974)* <u>Biochem.</u> *13:2822. Copyright by the American Chemical Society.]*

Table 2.   *REVERSAL OF AChR-^{3}H-TOXIN COMPLEX BY VARIOUS LIGANDS^a*

Ligand	Concn.(M)	Reversal(%)
Carbachol	0.01	25
	0.1	45
	0.5	73
Decamethonium	0.05	48
	0.1	48
d-Tubocurare	0.005	41
	0.05	61
N.n. siamensis neurotoxin	5×10^{-6}	23
	5×10^{-5}	56
α-bungarotoxin	5×10^{-6}	22
	5×10^{-5}	64
Lysozyme	1×10^{-4}	0
NaCl	0.5	0

^{a}^{3}H-toxin-AChR complex was prepared by incubating the standard assay mixture for one hour as described in Methods. Ligands were added to the reaction mixture to give the ligand concentrations listed and the reaction was incubated at room temperature for an additional hour. The final volume was 2.9 ml. The per cent reversal was determined by the decrease in precipitable counts compared to the assay without added ligand. ^{3}H-cobratoxin was present at 5×10^{-7} M. [Reprinted with permission from D.E. Ong and R.N. Brady (1974) *Biochem.* 13:2822. Copyright by the American Chemical Society.]

both the undissociated complex and the free AChR were retained by the resin. When the free AChR was eluted from the column with high salt and assayed for ^{3}H-cobratoxin-AChR complex formation (see Methods) it was verified that no AChR activity was lost during complex formation and reversal.

Affinity Chromatography. Although several neuroactive agents efficiently displace the toxin from the toxin-AChR complex when the complex is free in solution, once the toxin is covalently bound to the Sepharose matrix, reversal conditions change immensely. Dissociation studies were carried out using suspensions of toxin-bound Sepharose under incubation conditions of time, temperature, toxin concentrations, etc., similar to those employed for the dissociation studies of the free complex. Carbachol (0.5 M), decamethonium (0.3 M), d-tubocurare (0.02 M), formic acid (0.5 M), and sodium chloride (0.15 M), guanidine (6 M), mercaptoethanol (0.05 M), and dithioerythritol (0.05 M) were totally ineffective when employed to displace AChR from the absorbent-bound complex. Because of the inefficient AChR displacement in these batchwise experiments, a cycling system of continuous elution was designed (see Methods and Figure 1) to increase AChR yield. Carbachol (0.1 M) was selected as an eluent since a higher carbachol concentration precluded retention of the AChR protein on the DEAE Sephadex column.

Under the conditions employed, one cycle of the solubilized AChR preparation through the affinity column was sufficient to remove 90% of the available AChR activity. Further cycling of the same solubilized preparation never yielded greater than 96% adsorption even though the capacity of the column had not been exceeded. As noted earlier, approximately 10% of the immobilized cobratoxin retained the ability to bind AChR.

Recovery of free AChR from the DEAE-Sephadex column after continuous elution of the affinity column with 0.1 M carbachol is shown in Table 3. Approximately one-half of the bound AChR material is displaced by carbachol; the greatest portion being eluted within the first 24 hours. Recoveries of as high as 55% of bound AChR have been observed for a 24-hour elution.

Attempts to further purify the receptor protein by elution of the DEAE-Sephadex column with a step-wise gradient from 0.15 to 0.5 M sodium chloride (0.05 M steps) gave only a single protein peak, eluting between 0.2 and 0.3 M salt.

Table 3.   *RESULTS OF CONTINUOUS ELUTION OF SEPHAROSE-BOUND TOXIN-AChR COMPLEX WITH 0.1 M CARBACHOL AT 4°.*[a]

Time Period (hr.)	Recov. (% of bound AChR)	Equiv. Wt. (daltons)/ molecule of toxin bound
0-24	40.1	82,000
24-48	12.2	76,000
48-72	4.1	

[a]A solubilized preparation of excitable membrane protein was subjected to affinity chromatography as described in Methods. DEAE-Sephadex columns were removed after 24 hours and replaced with fresh columns. The isolated AChR was eluted from the DEAE-Sephadex (see Methods), and the per cent recovery and equivalent weight of the purified AChR were determined. Cycling solution was 0.1 M carbachol-0.01 M potassium phosphate-1% Triton X-100 (pH 7.0). [Reprinted with permission from D.E. Ong and R.N. Brady (1974) *Biochem.* 13:2822. Copyright by the American Chemical Society.]

Although different adsorbent preparations containing the same or different neurotoxins (cobratoxin, α-bungarotoxin, and *N.n. siamensis* neurotoxin) were essentially identical in capacity and percentage of active AChR-binding toxin molecules, some variation was observed in the efficiency with which AChR was eluted from batch to batch. Adsorbents which contained cobratoxin or *N.n. siamensis* neurotoxin yielded essentially the same percentage recovery; however, binding of the AChR to the α-bungarotoxin-Sepharose adsorbent was significantly more difficult to reverse. (Recovery of active AChR from these columns was approximately one-half that observed with the other two neurotoxins.)

The typical two-step purification procedure is described in Table 4. The isolated AChR protein has been purified 60-fold and has an equivalent weight of approximately 80,000 daltons per molecule of toxin bound. The acetylcholinesterase activity of this purified material is extremely low, representing about 0.005% by weight of the total recovered protein. High levels of acetylcholinesterase activity are present in the crude extract of the excitable membranes, but all the esterase activity applied to the affinity column is recovered in the nonadsorbed fractions.

If AChR protein is adsorbed to an affinity column and the adsorbent is eluted with several column volumes of 6M guanidine, the dialysed guanidine eluent contains protein but very little AChR activity. If such a guanidine-treated affinity column was inserted into the continuous elution system and eluted for 24 hours with 0.1M carbamylcholine, no protein or toxin-binding material was collected by the DEAE Sephadex column. Apparently the guanidine pretreatment eluted the AChR from the affinity column but irreversi-

Table 4. PURIFICATION OF ACETYCHOLINE RECEPTOR

Fraction	Protein (mg)	Act. (nmol of toxin bound)	Sp. Act. (nmol/mg)	Purifcn.-fold	Recov. (%)
Membrane suspension	35.2[a]	6.87	0.195		
Triton X-100 extract	17.6[a]	5.48	0.311	1.6	79.8
Purified receptor	0.242[b]	2.96	12.2	62	43.1

[a]By Lowry

[b]By amino acid analysis

[Reprinted with permission from D.E. Ong and R.N. Brady (1974) *Biochem.* 13:2822. Copyright by the American Chemical Society.]

bly denatured it in the process.

Gel Electrophoresis. The electrophoretic pattern of purified AChR protein isolated from an adsorbent containing as ligand *N.n. siamensis* neurotoxin is shown in Figure 4. In the presence of SDS, at least five polypeptide species are present, one band with an apparent molecular weight of 43,500, a grouping of three bands at molecular weights of 38,500, 35,500 and 33,500 and a major band observed at a position on the gel which indicates molecular weights greater than 70,000. This latter may represent multimers of the smaller species. Identical gel patterns were observed for AChR protein isolated from adsorbents utilizing α-bungarotoxin and cobratoxin as the adsorbing ligands (see Figure 5). When the protein fraction which was eluted from the affinity column by 6 M guanidine was examined by gel electrophoresis, an electrophoretic pattern identical with Figure 4 was obtained.

Amino Acid Composition. The preliminary amino acid compositions of AChR of *T. nobiliana*, *E. electricus* (Klett, Fulpius, Cooper, Smith, Reich, and Possani, 1973; Meunier, Sealock, Olsen, and Changeux, 1974), and *T. marmorata* (Eldefrawi and Eldefrawi, 1973; Heilbronn and Mattson, 1974) are given in Table 5. Each has a basic and acidic amino acid content of 11%-12% and 21%-23%, respectively, the latter of which does not include the amidated forms. Our results show the presence of tryptophan which was also found in the receptor from *T. marmorata* (Eldefrawi and Eldefrawi, 1973) and *E. electricus* (Meunier *et al.*, 1974). Noteworthy is the consistency and close agreement of the amino acid compositions of AChR from various species. At least over this limited phylogenetic spectrum, a common structure appears to have been preserved.

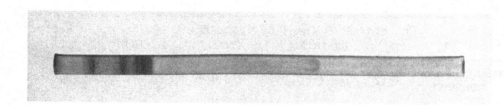

Figure 4. *Gel electrophoresis of purified AChR. AChR was purified by continuous elution affinity chromatography (see Methods) utilizing the neurotoxin of N.n. siamensis as ligand. Approximately 20 µg of the purified protein were electrophoresed as described in Methods. The gel was developed from left to right. [Reprinted from D.E. Ong and R.N. Brady (1974) Biochem. 13:2822. Copyright by the American Chemical Society.]*

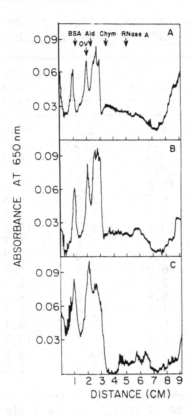

Figure 5. *Gel electrophoresis of purified AChR. AChR was puri-*
fied by continuous elution affinity chromatography
(see Methods) utilizing as ligands the neurotoxin of
N.n. siamensis (A), cobratoxin (B), and α-bungaro-
toxin (C). Approximately 20 μg of the purified AChR
were electrophoresed and scanned as noted in Methods.
[Reprinted with permission from D.E. Ong. and R.N.
Brady (1974) Biochem. 13:2822. Copyright by the
American Chemical Society.]

Due to the membranous environment of AChR *in vivo*, it is of
interest to determine its polarity and hydrophobic nature relative
to other proteins. Protein polarity has been estimated by the
percent of the polar residues asp, asn, glu, gln, lys, ser, arg,
thr, and his (Capaldi and Vanderkooi, 1972). By this criterion
the *T. nobiliana* AChR is 46% polar which is very similar to the
value of 47% reported for the *E. electricus* AChR (Meunier *et al.*,
1973). Analysis of a large number of proteins showed that most
of the soluble proteins had polarities of 47±6%, whereas many of
the membrane proteins had polarities less than 40% (Capaldi and

Table 5.   *AMINO ACID COMPOSITION* OF THE ACETYLCHOLINE RECEPTOR*
            PROTEIN FROM <u>*TORPEDO NOBILIANA*</u> *AND OTHER SPECIES*

	T. nobiliana	*T. marmorata*[a]	*T. marmorata*[b]	*E. electricus*[c]	*E. electricus*[d]
Lysine	4.5	6.1	5.0	4.6	6.3
Histidine	2.5	2.1	2.3	2.2	2.5
Arginine	3.7	3.5	3.7	4.2	4.2
Tryptophan	1.5	2.1	- +	0	2.4
Aspartic acid	12.2	11.8	12.5	11.4	9.8
Threonine	6.8	6.3	6.0	5.6	6.0
Serine	6.4	7.1	8.2	6.2	8.2
Glutamic acid	9.7	10.7	8.8	10.2	9.0
Proline	7.1	6.2	5.6	5.7	6.7
Glycine	5.0	6.4	5.0	5.9	4.8
Alanine	4.5	6.0	5.0	5.8	5.4
Half-cystine	2.8**	2.0	- ‡	2.0	1.7
Valine	6.2	5.5	7.5	8.6	6.9
Methionine	1.6	1.7	2.6	2.0	3.4
Isoleucine	6.2	5.2	7.5	6.4	8.1
Leucine	10.2	9.3	10.2	10.5	10.7
Tyrosine	4.2	3.6	3.7	4.0	3.8
Phenylalanine	4.2	4.4	4.6	5.7	5.1
Glucosamine	2.0	-	-	-	-

*The data are reported as mole%. It is a pleasure to thank
  Lilah Clack for the analysis of *T. nobiliana.*

**Represents the sum of half-cystine and cysteic acid.

+Not analyzed

‡Present but not quantitated.

[a]Eldefrawi and Eldefrawi (1973)

[b]Heilbronn and Mattson (1974)

[c]Klett *et al.* (1973)

[d]Meunier *et al.* (1974)
  (From Moore, Holladay, Puett, and Brady, 1974)

Vanderkooi, 1972). Using a somewhat more quantitative approach
involving transfer free energies (*e.g.*, from water to organic
solvent) of the various amino acid side chains (Goldsack, 1970;
Nozaki and Tanford, 1971), we find a hydrophobicity of 1236 cal
for the *T. nobiliana* AChR. This is only slightly greater than the

average value reported for several soluble proteins. For example, hemoglobin, cytochrome C, insulin, and lactic dehydrogenase have respective hydrophobicities of 1158, 1103, 1157, and 1127 ± 10% cal (Goldsack, 1970).

Glucosamine is present in the *T. nobiliana* AChR (about 3.8% w/w protein); however, the data are too tentative to conclude that AChR is a glycoprotein. Carbohydrate has also been reported in AChR of *E. electricus* (Meunier *et al.*, 1973) and hexosamine has been observed in *T. marmorata* (Eldefrawi and Eldefrawi, 1973), but its presence was attributed to an artifact arising from the affinity adsorption procedure.

Adsorption Spectroscopy. The ultraviolet adsorption spectrum of AChR is shown in Figure 6 and is characterized by an absorption maximum at 281 nm. The presence of tryptophan is clearly indicated from the spectrum by the shoulder at 290 nm and the shoulder at 260 nm is characteristic of phenylalanine.

Circular Dichroism Spectroscopy. The resolved (Zahler, Puett, and Fleisher, 1972) far ultraviolet circular dichroism spectrum of

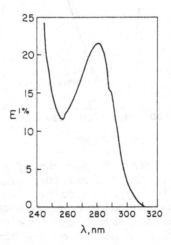

Figure 6. The adsorption spectrum of AChR in 0.1% Emulphogene BC-720 and the buffer described in the text. Light scattering corrections (e.g., A_{360}/A_{281} = 0.11) were made by extrapolating the apparent adsorbance (log A vs. log λ) between 320-360 nm to the region 240-320 nm. The protein concentration was taken as the average from amino-acid analysis and the Lowry method; agreement was within 1%. The absorbance at the 281 nm maximum for a 1% solution (1 cm) is 21.5. (From Moore, et al., 1974.)

AChR is shown in Figure 7. The spectrum between 205-245 nm is
characterized by two negative extrema at 207.5 and 215 nm with
mean residue ellipticities of -13,300 and -14,670 deg·cm²/dmole,
respectively. The spectrum can be fit to within ± 3% at all wave-
lengths by four resolved gaussian bands which are described in
Table 6. The 221 nm and 215 nm bands are assigned to the $n-\pi*$
transition of the peptide chromophore in α-helical regions and β-
structure, respectively. The lower wavelength bands probably

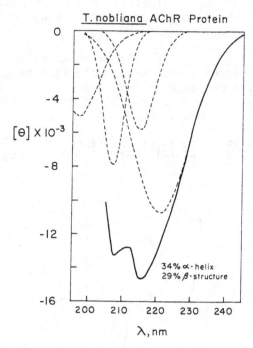

T. nobliana AChR Protein

34% α-helix
29% β-structure

*Figure 7.   The far ultraviolet CD spectrum of AChR (———) at ambi-
ent temperature and the resolved gaussian bands (- - -).
AChR was in the buffer containing 0.1% Emulphogene BC-
720. The experimental spectrum shown represents the
average of several sample and baseline scans. Repro-
ducibility was good and under the experimental conditions used (1.0 mm pathlength-fused silica cell, 3-
second time constant, and scale expansions of 2 milli-
degrees/inch and 7.5 nm/inch) the signal to noise ratio
was quite high, e.g., at 215 nm the baseline noise was
± 0.8 millidegrees and the signal was 14 ± 1 millidegrees. The mean residue ellipticity in units of deg·cm²
per dmole was calculated with a mean residue molecular
weight of 113.8 which was determined from the data in
Table 5 (Moore et al., 1974).*

Table 6.   *MEAN RESIDUE ROTATIONAL STRENGTHS OF THE FAR ULTRAVIOLET CIRCULAR DICHROIC BANDS OF THE T. NOBILIANA AChR AND MAJOR PROTEIN CONFORMERS*

AChR		Proteins[a]			
(λ_0, nm)	(R)[b]	(λ_0, nm)	(R)[b]	Transition	Conformer
221	-7.17	222	-21.0	n-π^*	α-helix
215	-1.99	215	- 7.77	n-π^*	β-structure
207	-2.11	208	- 6.26	π-π^*	α-helix
197	-2.47	197	- 7.27	π-π^*	aperiodic

[a]These data are from Puett, Ascoli, and Holladay (1974) and were resolved from the average CD spectra for the α-helical, β-structure, and aperiodic conformation as determined by Chen, Yang, and Martinez (1972).

[b]The rotational strength (R, in 10^{-42} cgs units) of each resolved gaussian band was obtained using the following relationship: $R \simeq (1.234 \times 10^{-42}) \cdot [\Theta°] \cdot \Delta/\lambda_0$, where $[\Theta°]$ and λ_0 denote the magnitude and wavelength of the extremum, and Δ is the bandwidth. (From Moore *et al.*, 1974.)

arise from the π-π^* transition of the peptide chromophore; however, the overlap of several large positive and negative bands in this region of the spectrum prohibits definitive resolution unless the experimental spectrum extends to about 185 nm.

We have used two methods (Robinson, Holladay, Picklesimer, and Puett, 1974) to estimate the type and amount of ordered secondary structure. One method involves a least-squares fit of AChR ellipticity from 207 to 243 nm to a linear combination of α-helical, β-structure, and aperiodic contributions (Chen *et al.*, 1972). The second method is based on a comparison of the rotational strengths of the 221 and 215 nm bands with the corresponding values (Puett *et al.*, 1974) for the pure conformers (Chen *et al.*, 1972).

These two methods gave the following values: 34% α-helix, 32% β-structure, and 34% aperiodic conformation by the least-squares analysis, and 35% α-helix, 26% β-structure, and thus 40% aperiodic conformation by the ratios of rotational strengths of the 221 and 215 nm bands. These results suggest that AChR contains a particularly high content of ordered secondary structure, *e.g.*, 34% α-helix and 29 ± 3% β-structure.

No attempt has been made to correct these estimates of second-

ary structure for the contributions of aromatic residues to the
far ultraviolet circular dichroism spectrum and for the effects of
light scattering. Generally, light scattering tends to reduce the
magnitude of the circular dichroism extrema (Zahler *et al.*, 1972)
and aromatic residues in model compounds exhibit positive ellipticity above about 215 nm (Holladay and Puett, unpublished). These
considerations lead to the conclusion that our estimates on the
amount of α-helix and β-structure probably represent minimal
values.

The effects of various cholinergic analogs on the circular
dichroism spectrum of AChR are currently under investigation.
Tentative data with carbamylcholine indicate that even low concentrations (*e.g.*, 1-4 μM which corresponds to low binding saturation)
alter both the magnitude of the apparent light scattering at 360 nm
and the circular dichroism spectrum in the vicinity of the 207.5 nm
extremum. These spectral changes noted at concentrations of the
ligand that are less than saturating levels give impetus to extending this work to saturating levels of the cholinergic ligand.

RESULTS--BRAIN

Binding of ^{125}I-α-bungarotoxin to Rat Brain Particulate Fraction. As indicated in Figure 8, the binding of ^{125}I-α-bungarotoxin
to a particulate fraction of whole rat brain appears to follow
typical Mechaelis-Menten kinetics. The process is saturable and
maximum binding occurred in the rage of 40-80 pmoles per gram protein (2-6 pmoles per gram original whole brain) depending on the
activity of the subcellular particles. Half saturation was reached at 8.3×10^{-9} M toxin. When particulate fractions from rat
liver (following the procedure used for brain) were incubated with
^{125}I-α-bungarotoxin under conditions identical to those described
for brain, no specific binding was detected.

The ability of various agents to inhibit toxin binding is
shown in Figure 9. D-Tubocurare, a nicotinic antagonist, is a
potent inhibitor, achieving 90% protection at 10^{-5} M. Atropine, a
potent muscarinic antagonist (inhibits muscarinic acetylcholine
receptors at 10^{-9} M), had little effect on binding at concentrations lower than 10^{-4} M. Similarly, eserine, an acetylcholinesterase inhibitor, and choline chloride reduced binding less than 10%
until concentrations greater than 10^{-4} M were present. Salt had
little effect on toxin binding even at high concentrations. Native α-bungarotoxin essentially abolished specific toxin-AChR binding at levels as low as 10^{-8} M.

The results of similar binding studies with solubilized membrane protein from excitable membranes of *T. nobiliana* are shown
in Figure 10. The inhibition pattern is very similar to that ob-

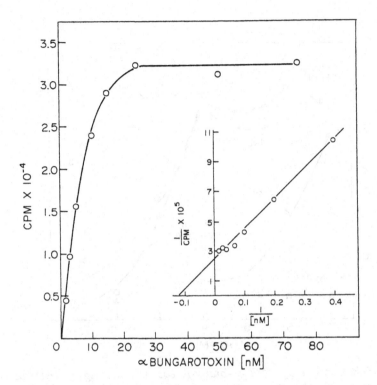

Figure 8. Binding of ^{125}I-α- bungarotoxin to a particulate fraction of rat brain. Five ml aliquots of the particu-
late fraction (see Methods) containing 5.8 mg protein/
ml (0.08 grams original brain weight/ml) were incubated in the presence of the indicated concentrations
of ^{125}I-α-bungarotoxin. Controls were run for each
concentration of ^{125}I-α-bungarotoxin by treating
samples with 2×10^{-6} M native α-bungarotoxin, prior
to addition of ^{125}I-α-bungarotoxin. Points shown on
the curve represent the difference between nonpretreated samples. The double reciprocal plot of the
data, shown in the insert, gave a value of $8.3 \times$
10^{-9} for half saturation.

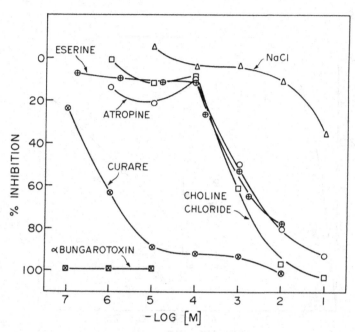

*Figure 9. Inhibition of ^{125}I-α-bungarotoxin binding to rat brain
particulate fractions. Whole rat brain particulate
fraction was obtained as described in Methods. Ten ml
aliquots of the particulate fraction containing 6.8 mg
protein/ml (0.09 grams original weight brain/ml) were
shaken for one hour at 23° with varying concentrations
of the above indicated agents. ^{125}I-α-bungarotoxin was
then added at a final concentration of 5 x 10^{-9} M and
incubation allowed to continue for one hour. The
amount of bound toxin was then obtained as described
in Methods. Controls were incubated with 10^{-6} native
α-bungarotoxin prior to addition of labeled toxin.
The per cent inhibition was determined by the decrease
in counts compared to nontreated samples.*

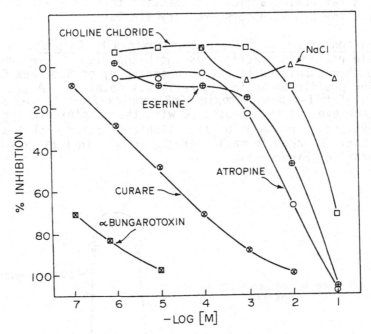

Figure 10. Inhibition of ^{125}I-α-bungarotoxin binding to a solubilized AChR preparation from <u>Torpedo nobiliana</u>. A
1% Emulphogene BC-720, 0.05 M sodium phosphate, pH
7.4 extract was prepared from the lyophilized electric organ of <u>T. nobiliana</u> as described by Ong and
Brady (1974). Samples containing soluble protein at
a concentration of 0.06 mg/ml were incubated with
shaking at 23° for one hour. The final volume of
1.0 ml contained 0.01 M sodium phosphate, 0.25%
Emulphogene BC-720 and the above indicated agents at
the stated concentrations. ^{125}I-α-bungarotoxin was
then added to a final concentration of 2.5 x 10^{-8} M
and incubation allowed to proceed for an additional
hour. At the end of the incubation period 5 ml of
0.25% Emulphogene, 0.01 M sodium phosphate, pH 7.4
were added to the assay solution. This solution
was filtered over Whatman DE-81 anion exchange
discs. Discs were washed with 15 ml of buffer and
counted in the γ-ray spectrometer. Controls were
run by incubating samples with 9.8 x 10^{-6} M native
α-bungarotoxin prior to ^{125}I-toxin addition. The
per cent inhibition was determined by the decrease
in counts compared to nontreated samples.

tained with rat brain particles suggesting that at least pharma-
cologically the two receptors are very similar.

    Formation of Brain ^{125}I-α-bungarotoxin-AChR Complex. When
the soluble rat brain fraction was incubated with ^{125}I-α-bungaro-
toxin and then submitted to gel chromatography of Sephadex G-100,
the elution profile shown in Figure 11 was obtained. A clean
separation of ^{125}I-α-bungarotoxin-AChR complex from ^{125}I-α-bungaro-
toxin is achieved by this procedure with the complex eluting in
the void volume. Treatment of the soluble fraction with 1 x 10^{-6}
α-bungarotoxin blocked formation of the ^{125}I-toxin AChR complex
(dotted profile, Figure 11).

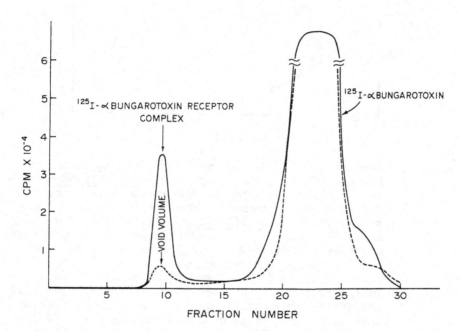

Figure 11.   Chromatography of solubilized brain ^{125}I-α-bungarotoxin-
AChR complex on Sephadex G-100. Rat brain particulate
fraction was solubilized as described in Methods. Ten
ml aliquots of the soluble fraction were incubated for
one hour at 23°C in the absence or presence of 10^{-6} M
native α-bungarotoxin. ^{125}I-α-bungarotoxin was then
added at a final concentration of 5 x 10^{-9} M and incubation continued for one hour. The nonpretreated (——)
and native (---) toxin pretreated samples were then
chromatographed separately on Sephadex G-100 columns
(2.5 x 32 cm). Fractions of 5.0 ml were collected and
radioactivity was determined.

As indicated in Figure 12, formation of the soluble ^{125}I-α-bungarotoxin AChR complex is saturable and demonstrates a value for half-saturation of 5×10^{-9} M ^{125}I-α-bungarotoxin.

The extent of complex formation is greatly decreased when either d-tubocurare, nicotine, carbachol, decamethonium, or native α-bungarotoxin are included in the assay mixture. As seen in Table 7, 10^{-5} M levels of nicotine and α-bungarotoxin abolish complex formation, whereas, carbachol, d-tubocurare, and decamethonium reduce ^{125}I-α-bungarotoxin-complex formation 35%-40% at similar concentrations. The neuroactive agents eserine (an acetylcholinesterase inhibitor), atropine and pilocarpine (muscarinic

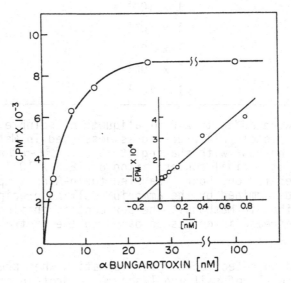

Figure 12.   Formation of brain ^{125}I-α-bungarotoxin-AChR complex. A soluble rat brain fraction was prepared as described in Methods. Two ml aliquots of the soluble fraction (6 mg protein/ml) were incubated with shaking for one hour at 23°C in the presence of ^{125}I-α-bungarotoxin at the indicated concentrations. Controls were run for each concentration of labeled toxin by pretreating the samples for an additional hour with 82.5 µg (5.2 x 10^{-6} M) native α-bungarotoxin prior to addition of labeled toxin. Formation of ^{125}I-α-bungarotoxin-receptor complex was measured by means of an ammonium sulfate precipitation assay (see Methods). The insert shows the double reciprocal plot of the data obtained and gives a half-saturation concentration for labeled toxin at 5.0 x 10^{-9} M.

Table 7.   INHIBITION OF BRAIN AChR-^{125}I-α-BUNGAROTOXIN COMPLEX
FORMATION BY VARIOUS LIGANDS[a]

Ligand	Concentration (M)	% Inhibition
α-bungarotoxin	1×10^{-5}	100
	1.7×10^{-6}	83
Nicotine	1×10^{-5}	100
Curare	1×10^{-5}	35
Carbachol	1×10^{-5}	37
Decamethonium	1×10^{-5}	40
Atropine	1×10^{-5}	0
Pilocarpine	1×10^{-5}	0
Eserine	1×10^{-5}	0
Lysozyme	1×10^{-5}	0
NaCl	1×10^{-1}	0

[a]Ligands were added to 2.0 ml aliquots of soluble rat brain
fraction (6 mg protein/ml) prepared as described in Methods, and
incubated for one hour with shaking at 23°C.   ^{125}I-α-bungarotoxin
was then added at a final concentration of 12.6×10^{-9} M and incubation continued for one hour.   Labeled toxin-AChR complex formation was then determined by the ammonium sulfate precipitation
assay as described in Methods.   The per cent inhibition was determined by the decrease in counts compared to the nontreated samples.

inhibitors) had no effect on complex formation when present at
10^{-5} M.   High levels of salt and lysozyme (a protein of low molecular weight and high pI) have no measurable effect on complex
formation.

As shown in Table 8, several detergents release the brain
AChR from its membrane matrix.   It is important to note that nonspecific binding sites (approximately 15%-20% of total binding)
are also solubilized and, hence, are present as contaminants in
the solubilized extract.   Emulphogene was selected for regular
usage because of its very low absorbance at 280 nm and its potential for use in spectroscopic studies.

Preparation of Horseradish Peroxidase-toxin Conjugate.   We
have recently coupled the α-toxin of N.n. siamensis to horseradish
peroxidase (HRP) by aldehyde coupling (Lutin, Jensen, Freeman, and
Brady, unpublished procedure).   The elution profiles of standard

Table 8. *EXTRACTION OF BRAIN* ^{125}I-α-*BUNGAROTOXIN-AChR COMPLEX*[a]

Detergent	% counts solubilized	
	nonprotected	Protected
1% v/v Triton X-100	78	
2% v/v Triton X-100	81	86
1% v/v Emulphogene BC-720	75	
2% v/v Emulphogene BC-720	76	89
1% w/v Lubrol WX	78	
2% w/v Lubrol WX	80	72

[a]Brain particulate receptor fractions were incubated with ^{125}I-α-bungarotoxin as described in Methods. Protected samples were incubated with 1×10^{-6} M native α-bungarotoxin prior to incubation with labeled toxin. Nonprotected samples were incubated only with labeled toxin. The resulting washed pellets containing bound ^{125}I-α-bungarotoxin were homogenized in 10 ml of 0.05 M sodium phosphate, pH 7.4, containing the above detergents at the indicated concentrations. These solutions were incubated with shaking as 23°C for two hours and then centrifuged at 34,800 x g for 30 minutes. Supernatants were removed and pellets were resuspended and counted to determine the per cent counts released.

HRP and neurotoxin (upper frame) and of a typical coupling reaction mixture (lower frame) are shown in Figure 13. HRP and toxin are completely separable and the reaction mixture profile suggests the presence of at least two new components.

The reaction products are extremely reproducible (see Figure 14) and the HRP-toxin conjugate retains both HRP activity and AChR binding capacity indefinitely.

Characterization of the HRP-toxin Conjugate. The dependence of HRP and HRP-toxin conjugate activities on pH is demonstrated in Figure 15. Since a potential contaminate of the HRP-toxin conjugate peak (Figure 14) is unreacted HRP the observation that the two curves are dissimilar is surprising. These two components are not separable in the system employed and, hence, the pH curves suggest the presence of only small amounts of unreacted HRP in the reaction mixture. Normal microscopic staining techniques employ HRP at pH 7.6, where its activity is at a maximum. The conjugate, interestingly, demonstrates little HRP activity at this pH. Staining techniques which utilize the conjugate will need to be modified accordingly.

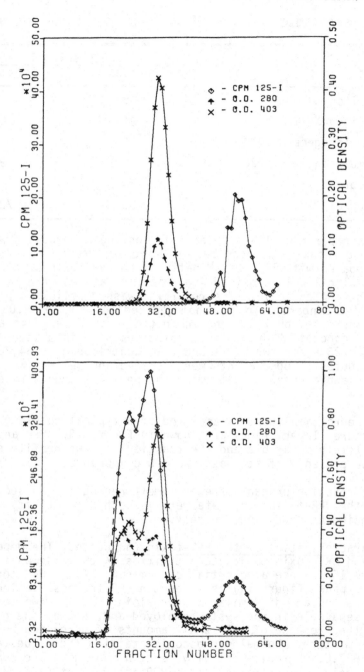

Figure 13. *Chromatography of HRP and N.n. siamensis (upper frame)*
and HRP-α-toxin aldehyde coupling reaction mixture
(lower frame) on Sephadex G-100.

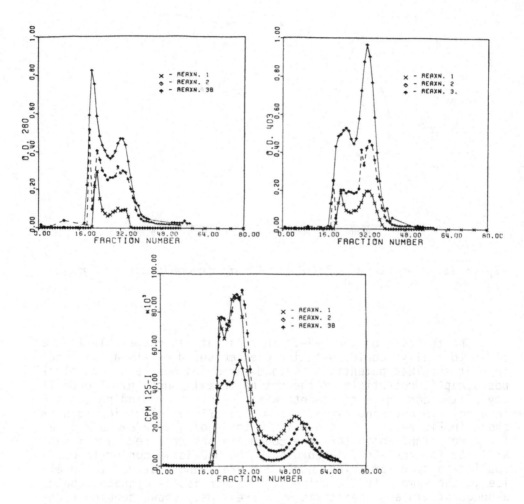

Figure 14. *Chromatography of HRP-α-toxin aldehyde coupling reaction on Sephadex G-100.*

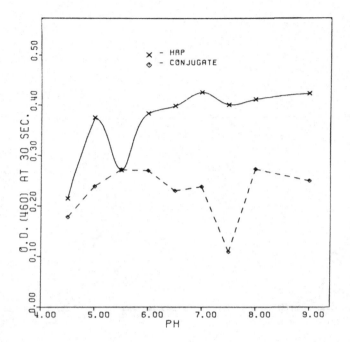

*Figure 15.   Dependence of HRP and HRP-toxin conjugate activities
on pH.*

        The toxicity of the HRP-toxin conjugate is comparable to that
of isotopically labeled α-toxins when measured by its ability to
inhibit endplate potentials in toad sartorius muscle and to block
postsynaptic potentials at the retino-tectal junction. The ability of the conjugate to compete with ^{3}H-toxin for binding to AChR
in a soluble membrane extract from *T. nobiliana* electric organ is
shown in Figure 16. Although the α-toxin of *N.n. siamensis* is a
far more potent inhibitor, the conjugate has retained significant
affinity for the AChR. Accordingly the HRP-toxin conjugate was
applied to toad sartorius muscle and brain and observed to localize in the same sites to which fluorescein isothiocyanate-labeled
α-bungarotoxin and ^{3}H-α-toxin were previously shown to bind (Jensen, Lutin, Freeman, and Brady, 1975).

                              DISCUSSION

        Successful application of affinity chromatography depends in
large part on how closely the experimental conditions permit the
ligand-protein interaction to simulate the reactions observed when
the components are free in solution. Examination of the amino

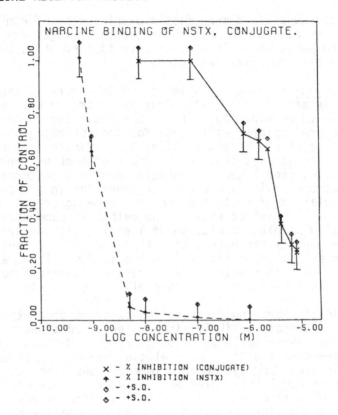

Figure 16.   Inhibition of AChR-³H-toxin complex formation by HRP-toxin conjugate and native α-toxin of N.n. siamensis.

acid sequences of the three neurotoxins employed as ligands, shows that each had a lysine residue which is in close proximity to one of the residues thought to play a central role in toxin-AChR inter-action (Harrington and Brady, unpublished data).   Hence, covalent linkage to the Sepharose resin through the ε-amino group of this lysine would probably preclude formation of the toxin-AChR com-plex.   Chang, Yang, Nakai, and Hayashi (1971) reported that this same lysine is the most reactive lysine in the cobratoxin molecule; predominant coupling of the toxin to the resin through this resi-due would explain the observation that only 10% of the toxin mole-cules retain the ability to bind to AChR after they are coupled to the Sepharose.   It is also apparent that covalent linkage of the toxin-AChR complex to the Sepharose significantly changes the ligand-protein interactions since displacement of the AChR is more readily accomplished when the complex is free in solution.   Recent-ly, efforts were made to introduce a "bridge" between the toxin and resin in order to produce more facile displacement of AChR. These efforts were successful in that a six-carbon "bridge" was introduced with no perceivable loss of ability to bind AChR, but no increase in complex reversal was noted.

Receptor Purification. As indicated in Figure 4, isolation of the AChR by affinity chromatography as described herein does not give rise to a unique polypeptide species. The three neurotoxins which are employed as ligands for the chromatography vary in amino acid content, molecular size, and affinity for the AChR. That the protein species isolated by means of each of these immobilized toxins (see Figure 5) exhibit identical patterns upon SDS gel electrophroesis is a strong argument for the concept that a unique population of protein molecules is being selectively isolated. The high selectivity of the method is demonstrated by the essentially complete exclusion of acetylcholine esterase from the adsorbent and by the observation that only AChR protein binds to the adsorbent since elution with 6 M guanidine yields a protein fraction with an electrophoretic pattern identical to that obtained by elution with 0.1 M carbachol, a cholinergic ligand.

Contamination arising from the ion-exchange properties in the resin is extremely unlikely since material adsorbed to the column in this manner would be removed by the 1 M sodium chloride wash which precedes the continuous elution process. Although impurities resulting from hydrophobic interactions with the adsorbent can not be completely ruled out, they are highly unlikely since their appearance would require the specific reversal of the hydrophobic interactions by 0.1 M carbachol, a cholinergic ligand. A possible explanation for the presence of more than one molecular species in our preparation is receptor multiplicity. Plurality of binding sites has been reported for two species of *T. nobiliana* (Eldefrawi, Eldefrawi, Gilmour, & O'Brien, 1971; Raftery, Schmidt, and Clark, 1972) and heterogeneity on SDS gels has been previously observed for material purified by affinity chromatography employing covalently-bound quaternary ammonium functions as ligands (Schmidt and Raftery, 1973). Purified α-bungarotoxin-AChR complex, obtained by using α-bungarotoxin to displace AChR from an affinity column containing cobratoxin as ligand, shows heterogeneity after SDS electrophoresis (Raftery, 1973). As in the present study, the major species are in the 35,000-45,000 molecular weight range.

A third, and as yet unconsidered, explanation of the heterogeneity is the concept that the AChR protein is tightly associated in the membrane with specific nontoxin-binding proteins. Treatment with Triton X-100 might lead to cosolubilization such that the integrity of the protein-protein interactions is undisturbed. The associated proteins could be carried through the affinity chromatography purification and eluted from the DEAE-Sephadex column still attached to the AChR. Treatment for SDS gel electrophoresis would then disrupt the association and upon electrophoresis this specific population of nontoxin-binding proteins would be revealed.

The most likely possibility, however, is that the several species observed upon SDS gel electrophoresis are a result of proteolytic hydrolysis of the AChR protein while in the crude solubilized preparation or during the extended period of time required for the affinity chromatography.

An equivalent weight of 80,000 daltons/molecule of toxin bound is consistently obtained by this procedure; a value which is in harmony with data from several other laboratories (Karlin, 1974). Since the majority of isolated protein falls in the molecular weight range of 33,000-43,000 unless more than one toxin molecule binds to a single polypeptide, the lowest equivalent weight possible would probably also be in this range. Since we observe four species of approximately equal quantity in this range, an equivalent weight of 80,000 would appear to require that some of the species not bind toxin. We observed a single peak of purified AChR in the molecular weight range greater than 200,000 when the material was applied to a calibrated Sephadex G-200 column.

The AChR appears to be a major constituent of the electroplax membrane protein. Based on an equivalent weight of 80,000 daltons, the 60-fold purification suggests that as much as 1.5% of membrane protein is AChR.

The *T. nobiliana* AChR has gross polarity and hydrophobicity characteristics like those of many soluble proteins. Unfortunately, these considerations provide no information on the distribution of hydrophobic residues. The portion of AChR containing the cholinergic-binding site is most certainly located on the membrane surface and exposed to the synaptic cleft. However, the solubility properties of AChR indicate extensive hydrophobic regions and, thus, part of the AChR may penetrate the membrane. It is of immense interest to determine if the hydrophilic and hydrophobic residues are randomly distributed along the polypeptide backbone or are clustered in distinct regions. The answer to this important issue must await additional chemical studies.

Our finding of a high content of ordered secondary structure in AChR is of interest both in assessing the conformation of AChR and in comparative conformational studies. For example, other studies have shown that the average α-helicity of mitrochondrial membrane proteins is about 27% and there is not a large amount of β-structure (Zahler *et al.*, 1972). Also, they found that the intrinsic mitochondrial membrane proteins are more helical than the extrinsic proteins.

Frequently, β-structure in proteins is associated with a relatively compact structural core and, thus, much of AChR may exist in an extensively folded conformation (*i.e.*, globular-like) reminiscent of soluble proteins. Indeed, the electron micrographs of AChR tend to support this model (Cartaud, Benedetti, Cohn, Meunier, and Changeux, 1973; Meunier, Sugiyama, Cartaud, Sealock, and Changeux, 1973).

Many speculations can be made regarding the role and locations of the α-helical and β-structure regions. For example, the α-helical regions may exhibit conformational amphipathic properties (Assman and Brewer, 1973; Segrest, Jackson, Morrisett, and Gotto, 1974) in which hydrophilic side-chains are located mainly on one surface area of an α-helix while the other is comprised primarily of hydrophobic side-chains. An array of such structures within the ionophore would constitute an excellent ion channel from a thermodynamic viewpoint since the hydrophobic groups would be in contact with an aqueous phase and the hydrophonic groups would be located within an apolar environment arising either from the protein or the lipid moiety. Regions of β-structure may, of course, be involved in forming the ion channel, but it would seem that their predominant location would be within the globular portions of the protein.

The binding of ^{125}I-α-bungarotoxin to particulate fractions from rat brain suggests the presence of a nicotinic acetylcholine receptor in this tissue. This observation is strongly supported by the ligand-binding characteristics of the solubilized toxin-binding component.

Our results indicate a concentration of nicotinic-binding sites of 10^{-14} M per milligram of protein. Based on this value one can conservatively calculate that 1,000 g of lyophilized brain would contain approximately 0.5 mg of acetylcholine receptor protein (based upon a molecular weight of 80,000 daltons for the receptor). At these concentrations, only a highly selective affinity chromatography system would appear to afford a feasible method for the isolation of AChR from mammalian tissue since, at these levels, purification by classical procedures would seem to be impossible. Affinity chromatography utilizing snake neurotoxins as ligands appears to provide such selectivity. However, since the normal yield from these columns is often low (15%-20%), more efficient methods must be developed. One such alternative is shown in Figure 17. ω-amino alkyl-Sepharose can be prepared by reacting diamine derivatives, $NH_2(CH_2)_n-NH_2$, with cyanogen bromide-activated Sepharose. Very little crosslinking occurs if a large excess of diamine is used, so that it is relatively easy to insert extensions of considerable length. The amino-Sepharose derivative can be treated with *p*-nitrobenzoyl azide in 50% dimethylformamide, reduced to the aminophenyl derivative with sodium dithionite, and

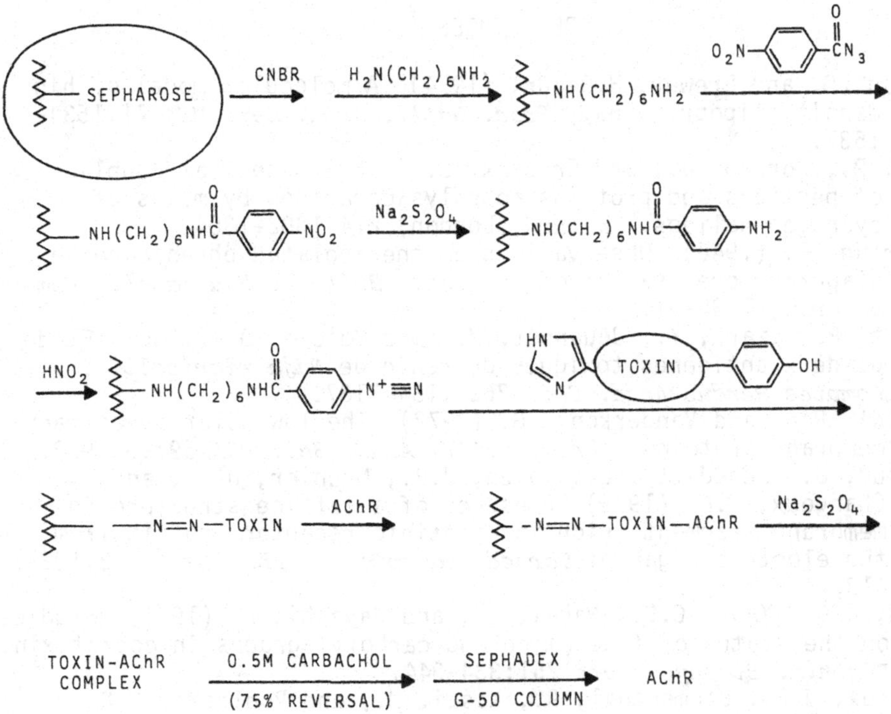

Figure 17. Isolation of AChR by affinity chromatography with azo-linked ligands.

diazotized with nitrous acid. Ligands having phenolic or imidazole groups (the neurotoxin) react rapidly with diazonium-Sepharose. A special advantage of these azo-linked ligands is the susceptibility to cleavage of the ligand-Sepharose bond by reduction with 0.1 M sodium dithionite at pH 8. Thus, through azo linkage the neurotoxin can be coupled to Sepharose and then, after selective adsorption of the receptor, the complex can be removed intact from the Sepharose by treatment with sodium dithionite. Once cleaved, the complex can be reversed while free in solution and passed over Sephadex G-50 to separate AChR from toxin. The isolated AChR from brain could then be studied extensively. Such experiments are currently underway in our laboratory.

REFERENCES

Assman, G. and Brewer, H.B. Jr. (1974) A molecular model of high density lipoproteins. *Proc. Nat'l. Acad. Sci. USA* **71**:1534-1537.

Axen, R., Porath, J., and Ernback, S. (1967) Chemical coupling of peptides and proteins to polysaccharides by means of cyanogen halides. *Nature* (London) **214**:1302-1304.

Bülbring, E. (1946) Observations on the isolated phrenic nerve diaphragm preparation of the rat. *Brit. J. Pharmacol. Chemotherapy* **1**:38-61.

Boquet, P., Izard, Y., Jouannet, M., and Meaume, J. (1966) Etude de deux antigènes toxiques du renin de *Naja nigricollis*. *Comptes Rendus Acad. Sci.* **262**:1134-1137.

Capaldi, R.A. and Vanderkooi, G. (1972) The low polarity of many membrane proteins. *Proc. Nat'l. Acad. Sci. USA* **69**:930-932.

Cartaud, J., Benedetti, L., Cohen, J.B., Meunier, J.C., and Changeux, J.P. (1973) Presence of a lattice structure in membrane fragments rich in nicotinic receptor protein from the electric organ of *Torpedo marmorata*. *FEBS Lett.* **33**:109-113.

Chang, C.C., Yang, C.C., Nakai, K., and Hayashi, K. (1971) Studies on the status of free amino and carboxyl groups in cobratoxin. *Biochim. Biophys. Acta* **251**:334-344.

Changeux, J.P., Blumenthal, R., Kasai, M., and Podleski, T.R. (1970) Conformational transitions in the course of membrane excitation. In: *Molecular properties of drug receptors* (R. Porter and J. O'Conner, eds.) pp. 197-217, CIBA Foundation Symposium, Churchill, London.

Chen, Y., Yang, J.R., and Martinez, H.M. (1972) Determination of the secondary structures of proteins by circular dichroism and optical rotary dispersion. *Biochemistry* **11**:4120-4131.

deRobertis, E. and Schacht, J. (eds.) (1974) *Neurochemistry of cholinergic receptors*. Raven Press, New York.

Eldefrawi, M.E. and Eldefrawi, A.J. (1973) Purification and molecular properties of the acetylcholine receptor from *Torpedo* electroplax. *Arch. Biochem. Biophys.* **159**:362-372.

Eldefrawi, M.E., Eldefrawi, A.J., Gilmour, L.R., and O'Brien, R.D. (1971) Multiple affinities for binding of cholinergic ligands to a particulate fraction of *Torpedo* electroplax. *Mol. Pharmacol.* **7**:420-427.

Ellman, G.L., Courtney, K.D., Andres, V., and Featherstone, R. (1961) A new and rapid colorimetric determination of acetylcholinesterase activity. *Biochem. Pharmacol.* **7**, 88-95.

Franklin, G.I. and Potter, L.T. (1972) Studies of the binding of α-bungarotoxin to membrane-bound and detergent-dispersed acetylcholine receptors from *Torpedo* electric tissue. *FEBS Lett.* **28**:101-106.

Goldsack, D.E. (1970) Relation of the hydrophobicity index to the thermal stability of homologous proteins. *Biopolymers* **9**:247-252.

Heilbronn, E. and Mattson, C. (1974) The nicotinic cholinergic
    receptor protein: Improved purification method, preliminary
    amino acid composition and observed auto-immuno response. *J.
    Neurochem*. 22:315-316.

Jensen, C.F., Lutin, W.A., Freeman, J.A., and Brady, R.N. Localiza-
    tion of acetylcholine receptor in brain using horseradish per-
    oxidase conjugated snake neurotoxin. *Proc. Am. Soc. Cell
    Biol*., in press.

Karlin, A. (1967) Permeability and internal concentration of ions
    during depolarization of the electroplax. *Proc. Nat'l. Acad.
    Sci. USA* 58:1162-1167.

Katz, B. (1966) *Nerve, muscle and synapse*. McGraw Hill, New York.

Klett, R.P., Fulpius, B.W., Cooper, D., Smith, M., Reich, E., and
    Possani, L.D. (1973) The acetylcholine receptor, purifica-
    tion and characterization of a macromolecule isolated from
    Electrophorus electricus. *J. Biol. Chem*. 248:6841-6853.

Lee, C.Y. and Chang, C.C. (1966) Modes of action of purified
    toxins from elapid venoms on neuromuscular transmissions.
    Mem. Inst. Butanan, San Paulo, 33:555-572.

Liu, T.Y. and Chang, Y.H. (1971) Hydrolysis of proteins with p-
    toluenesulfonic acid determination of tryptophan. *J. Biol.
    Chem*. 246:2842-2848.

Lowry, O.H., Rosebrough, N.J., Farr, A.L., and Randall, R.J. (1951)
    Protein measurement with the Folin phenol reagent. *J. Biol.
    Chem*. 193:265-275.

Meunier, J.C., Sealock, R., Olsen, R., and Changeux, J.P. (1974)
    Purification and properties of the cholinergic receptor pro-
    tein from *Electrophorus electricus* electric tissue. *Eur. J.
    Biochem*. 45:371-394.

Meunier, J.C., Sugiyama, H., Cartaud, J., Sealock, R., and Changeux,
    J.P. (1973) Functional properties of the purified cholinergic
    receptor protein from *Electrophorus electricus*. *Brain Res*.
    62:307-315.

Moore, W.M., Holladay, L.A., Puett, D., and Brady, R.N. (1974) On
    the conformation of the acetylcholine receptor protein from
    Torpedo nobiliana. *FEBS Lett*. 45:145-149.

Morrison, M. and Bayse, G.S. (1970) Catalysis of iodination by
    lactoperoxidase. *Biochemistry* 9:2995-3000.

Nachmansohn, D. (1959) *Chemical and molecular basis of nerve
    activity*. Academic Press, New York.

Nozaki, Y. and Tanford, C. (1971) The solubility of amino acids
    and two glycine peptides in aqueous ethanol and dioxane solu-
    tions. *J. Biol. Chem*. 246:2211-2217

Ong, D.E. and Brady, R.N. (1974) Isolation of cholinergic receptor
    protein(s) from *Torpedo nobiliana* by affinity chromatography.
    Biochemistry 13:2822-2827.

Puett, D., Ascoli, M., and Holladay, L.A. (1974) Conformational
    and metabolic aspects of gonadotropins. In: *Hormone binding
    and target cell activation in the testis*, Vol. I Current
    topics in molecular endocrinology (A.R. Means and M.L. Dufau,

eds.), pp. 109-124, Plenum Press, New York.

Raftery, M.A. (1973) Isolation of acetylcholine receptor-α-bungarotoxin complexes from *Torpedo californica* electroplax. *Arch. Biochem. Biophys.* 154:270-276.

Raftery, M.A., Schmidt, J., and Clark, P.G. (1972) Specificity of α-bungarotoxin binding to *Torpedo californica* electroplax. *Arch. Biochem. Biophys.* 152:882-886.

Rang, H.P. (ed.) (1973) *Drug receptors.* University Park Press, Baltimore.

Reisfeld, R.A., Lewis, U.J., and Williams, D.E. (1962) Disk electrophoresis of basic proteins and peptides on polyacrylamide gels. *Nature* (London) 195:281-283.

Rice, R.H. and Means, G.E. (1971) Radioactive labeling of proteins *in vitro*. *J. Biol. Chem.* 246, 831-832.

Robinson, J.P., Holladay, L.A., Picklesimer, J.B., and Puett, D. (1974) Tetanus toxin conformation. *Mol Cell. Biochem.* 5: 147-151.

Schmidt, J. and Raftery, M.A. (1973) A simple assay for the study of solubilized acetylcholine receptors. *Anal. Biochem.* 52:349-354.

Segrest, J.P., Jackson, R.L., Morrisett, J.D., and Gotto, A.M. Jr. (1974) A molecular theory lipid-protein interactions in the plasma lipoproteins. *FEBS Lett.* 38:247-253.

Shih, J.W. and Hash, J.H. (1971) The N, O-diacetylmuramidase of Chalaropsis species. *J. Biol. Chem.* 246:994-1006.

Weber, K.and Osborn, M. (1969) The reliability of molecular weight determinations by dodecyl sulfate-polyacrylamide gel electrophoresis. *J. Biol. Chem.* 244:4406-4412.

Yang, C.C. (1964) Purification of toxic proteins from cobra venom. *Tai-Wan I Hsueh Hui Tsa Chih* 63:325.

Zahler, W.L., Puett, D., and Fleischer, S. (1972) Circular dichroism of mitochondrial membranes before and after extraction of lipids and surface proteins. *Biochim. Biophys. Acta* 255:365-379.

ACKNOWLEDGEMENT

Appreciation is extended to Miss Katy Welch for her excellent assistance. This study was supported, in part, by USPHS grants NS-11439 and MH-08107.

DISCUSSION AFTER DR. BRADY'S PAPER

Dr. Hechter
    I have a series of short, technical questions. With respect to your best *Torpedo* receptor preparation of molecular weight about 200,000, do you have a homogeneous protein?

Dr. Brady
    Yes.

Dr. Hechter
    You've indicated that this protein has carbohydrate. How much?

Dr. Brady
    It appears to be in the neighborhood of 3%-4% w/w protein.

Dr. Hechter
    Does this receptor preparation have any lipid? Does extraction with chloroform-methanol-acid remove lipid?

Dr. Brady
    The purified receptor protein from the affinity columns does not contain any lipid.

Dr. Hechter
    Measured how?

Dr. Brady
    By staining techniques.

Dr. Hechter
    Did you detect one molecule of phospholipid per molecule of receptor?

Dr. Brady
    No, we didn't.

Dr. Hechter
    Well, could your techniques detect that?

Dr. Brady
    Yes, and we didn't detect any at all.

Dr. Hechter
    I'm sure you know that deRobertis has prepared proteolipid fractions with chloroform-methanol extraction which he feels contains cholinergic receptors. Would you comment on the deRobertis approach to the acetylcholine receptor?

Dr. Brady
    I'd be glad to comment on that. It's interesting. When we
initially started working with the purification, we tried to repeat the chloroform-methanol extracts, and we were unable to repeat deRobertis' work. I do know that other laboratories have
tried to do the same thing and, of course, if that particular procedure could be verified it would be advantageous because one
could extract one time with chloroform-methanol and have purified
cholinergic receptor protein. The properties reported, molecular
weights, etc. for the cholinergic proteolipid are very similar to
those reported for detergent extracted receptor. I think the best
thing to say is that we're just unable to reproduce this data. We
have a very difficult time with the LH-20 columns. I don't know
why. We seem to be unable to wash them clean. No matter how much
we wash the columns, when we start an elution we get peaks. Now,
I know that other laboratories have tried and have also been un-
successful. deRobertis is successful, and that's all I care to
comment about it. With respect to the black lipid membranes,
Bernard at SUNY and Goodall at Alabama have extracted these receptors with detergents and applied them to black lipid bilayers.
They've been successful. It should also be remembered, however,
that Mahler has been successful with similar experiments in which
the esterase was reconstituted back into the lipid bilayers and
they observed similar conductance changes associated with them,
so until these conductance changes can be demonstrated to be very
specific and that the conductance changes are associated with
specific ion translocations, it's hard to draw definitive conclusions. An excellent experiment would be to extract with chloroform-methanol and then to perform dialysis procedures designed to
transfer the receptor protein from the organic solvents to an
aqueous medium. Theoretically, you ought to end up with the same
receptor, but nobody's done these experiments successfully; many
have tried.

Dr. Lefkowitz
    I have a very simple question. I was wondering what the spe-
cific radioactivities of the tritiated toxins and the iodinated
toxins are that you're talking about, and why you switched to
iodinated bungarotoxin for the rat brain whereas you had been
using a tritiated toxin earlier.

Dr. Brady
    Our original specific activities were approximately two curies
per millimol with cobratoxin. When we went to the *N.n. siamensis*
neurotoxin the specific activity increased to eight curies per millimol because there are more lysines in this polypeptide. We make
a dimethyllysine derivative of the toxin. We like this derivative
because it doesn't significantly change the charge on the molecule
and, therefore, causes less changes in conformation. The specific
activity of the iodide is approximately 30 curies per millimol.

The eight curies per millimol is marginal for what we want to do, but we don't have any problems with the iodide.

Dr. Lefkowitz
   So, in other words, for the brain, where there are many less sites, you needed higher specific activity.

Dr. Brady
   That's correct. Last summer Dr. Changeux and I had a discussion concerning the receptor in brain. He indicated they had not seen any activity, and I suggested that the specific activity of his toxin might be too low. When we went to the higher specific activity, we began to see receptor activity in brain.

Dr. Lefkowitz
   Did the specific activity he was using to conclude that they weren't there below the levels you used?

Dr. Brady
   It was in the range of eight to ten curies per millimol; in that neighborhood, which is very marginal.

Dr. Hechter
   If you take an aqueous solution of your purified acetylcholine receptor and add two volumes of chloroform, one volume of methanol, and shake it up, do you get denatured protein at the interface?

Dr. Brady
   We haven't done that.

Dr. Hechter
   That's what happens when you work with most proteins. If there is a proteolipid, something should be present in the chloroform-methanol phase.

Dr. Brady
   That's correct.

Dr. Hechter
   Has anybody done this experiment?

Dr. Brady
   Potter has, and he suggests it did not work. The only thing that I've ever seen on this was a report that he made at a symposium where he remarked that he'd tried it and it hadn't worked.

Dr. Black
   I have a comment and then a question. We're interested in the superior cervical ganglion, which contains both nicotinic cholinergic and muscarinic cholinergic synapses. The differences between

these two cholinergic synapses are rather remarkable. The nicotinic cholinergic receptor on the principal ganglionic neuron generates a fast excitatory postsynaptic potential which has a half
millisecond latency. Conductance changes and increased ion flux
are involved in the generation of the fast excitatory postsynaptic
potential by the nicotinic cholinergic receptor, while the muscarinic cholinergic receptor generates a slow excitatory postsynaptic potential, with a 200 to 300 millisecond latency. Increased
membrane excitatory postsynaptic potential is apparently involved
with decreased ion flow if anything, although that's controversial.
The muscarinic cholinergic receptor is apparently linked to a
guanylate cyclase, so that activation of the muscarinic cholinergic receptor causes increased cyclic GMP generation (Kebabian,
Steiner, and Greengard, 1975; Weight, Petzold, and Greengard,
1975). My question is, is anyone pursuing the isolation of the
muscarinic cholinergic receptor from nervous tissue?

Dr. Brady
     Yes they are. The problem is the same problem as described
by Dr. Lefkowitz earlier. We do not have a ligand to isolate receptor in the concentration of 10^{-14} molar binding sites per gram
of protein. There is a specific ligand developed by the military,
QNB, that Snyder's lab has used to characterize the muscarinic
receptor.

Dr. Black
     I was just pointing out that one could use the presence of
the guanylate cyclase to monitor activity of the muscarinic cholinergic receptor, just as Dr. Lefkowitz is using the adenylate
cyclase to monitor the β-adrenergic receptor.

Dr. Brady
     Perhaps.

Dr. Forte
     Has it ever been shown that the guanylate cyclase is coupled
to that receptor analogous to the adenylate cyclase and catecholamine?

Dr. Brady
     Yes, it's pretty obvious. The characterization of this sys-
tem is not beyond the pharmacological stage at this time.

Dr. Forte
     That's true; I've never seen the sort of evidence that would
really link the two together. There is presumptive evidence that
if you put in a muscarinic agonist that you might see an increase
in cell levels of cyclic GMP, but that doesn't mean they're coupled,
not in the concept of catalytic unit coupled to a regulatory receptor subunit.

Dr. Lefkowitz
Yes, I was going to say that. I think Dr. Forte's point is
really well taken. I don't think anybody would argue that there
are a number of pharmacological systems in which you can show that
muscarinic cholinergic agents elevate cyclic GMP levels. To my
knowledge, and Dr. White might want to comment on this, all direct
attempts to show that cholinergic agonists stimulate guanylate
cyclase in analogy with adrenergic agents stimulating adenylate
cyclase have failed.

Dr. Brady
Let me add one additional comment concerning the involvement
of lipids that Dr. Hechter has already commented on. When you
solubilize the receptor from electroplaques, you require some
kind of detergent, and that detergent is required in the purification procedure, but when you eventually end up with the purified
material, the requirement for the detergent is lost. It's also
interesting that, when you do kinetics on the purified receptor,
the binding properties of the receptor have been modified in the
purification procedure, and the affinity for the cholinergic ligands is actually greater in the purified receptor than it is in
crude preparations of electroplaques membranes.

Dr. Hechter
How many detergent molecules are associated with receptor
molecules?

Dr. Brady
There are many. It is calculated that 200-250 detergent molecules are associated with each receptor molecule. In essence,
it's a proteo-detergent.

Dr. Hechter
So you really haven't removed lipid?

Dr. Brady
We've just replaced it with detergent, right.

Dr. Forte
The receptor protein from the electroplaques, though, was
not soluble after detergent removal, after purification?

Dr. Brady
It depends on which laboratory says that. Changeux says that
his is, and he doesn't require detergent after he purifies it.
Reich also said the detergent requirement is eliminated once the
receptor is pure.

Dr. Hechter
The differences cited may relate to how much detergent re-

mains associated with the protein, after treatments designed to
remove detergent from the preparation. It is very difficult to
remove all of the detergent molecules.

Dr. Brady
     That's correct. After purification, the number of detergent
molecules associated with the receptor is sufficient to keep it in
solution and you don't require detergent in your buffers and
other materials.

Dr. Campbell
     In your investigation of the polarity of the complex from
amino acid composition you didn't indicate the percentage of
amides in aspartic and glutamic residues. Do you know that?

Dr. Brady
     No, we did not use them in those calculations.

Dr. Sun
     In one of your slides you have shown the CD of the purified
receptor. Did you see any change before and after the binding of
bungarotoxin or coupled to bungarotoxin?

Dr. Brady
     We looked at this to see if we could show any changes in
secondary structure with carbachol and were unable to do so. In
the beginning we were very disappointed by this, but the more we
thought about it the more we realized that those changes would be
associated with tertiary structure and not secondary structure,
so that it wasn't surprising that we weren't able to see any. Our
intention now, of course, is to isolate milligram quantities of
the receptor and to seek perturbations of the tryptophan environment.

Dr. Hechter
     If you were to put labelled bungarotoxin into your purified
Torpedo receptor, wash out all excess bungarotoxin, and then take
the complex and put it into SDS, would the bungarotoxin be located
in one of the specific subunits?

Dr. Brady
     The problem is that the SDS dissociates totally the toxin
from either subunit, and when you do that experiment you see a 50
and a 42, and then you see α-bungarotoxin down at the bottom of
the gel. It completely dissociates from the receptor in SDS.

Dr. Hechter
     Is it possible to split the complex with a gentler detergent,
so that you can get subunits, without having to use SDS?

Dr. Brady
    We haven't done that. We'd like to find a mechanism to
demonstrate which of the bands the toxin associates itself with,
but to date we haven't been able to do this. SDS is the only
agent that we've looked at extensively and it dissociates the
complex completely.

DISCUSSION REFERENCES

Kebabian, J.W., Steiner, A.L., and Greengard, P. (1975) Muscarinic
    cholinergic regulation of cyclic guanosine 3'-5'-monophos-
    phate in autonomic ganglia: Possible role in synaptic trans-
    mission. *J. Pharmacol. Exp. Ther.* 193:474-488.
Weight, F.F., Petzold, G., and Greengard, P. (1974) Guanosine
    3',5'-monophosphate in sympathetic ganglia: Increase associ-
    ated with synaptic transmission. *Science* 186:942-944.

INSULIN BINDING BY CULTURED FIBROBLASTS FROM NORMAL AND INSULIN-RESISTANT SUBJECTS

A.L. Rosenbloom,* S. Goldstein, and C.C. Yip

Departments of Medicine, Biochemistry, and Pediatrics
McMaster University, Hamilton, Ontario
Banting and Best Institute of the University of Toronto

The major advantage of cultured fibroblasts (CF) for the study of genetic regulatory aspects of insulin binding is the unrestricted use of stable diploid human cells several generations removed from neuro-humoral influences. CF were grown to confluence in 100 mm plastic dishes, 6-10 subcultures after harvesting from skin explants. Donors included 11 nondiabetic controls aged three months to 70 years, four children two to nine years old with precocious tissue degeneration--three with Progeria (Rosenbloom and DeBusk, 1971) and one with Rothmund-Thomson Syndrome (Blinstrub, Lehman, and Steinberg, 1964)--and three persons ages 15, 19, and 30 years with lipoatrophic diabetes (LD). LD is a condition characterized by extremely high circulating insulin levels and resistance to the effects of massive doses of injected insulin (Flier, Kahn, Roth, and Bar, 1975).

After washing adherent cells, 1.2 ml medium containing 1% albumin, 20 mM Hepes buffer, pH 7.0, ^{125}I-insulin, labeled using lactoperoxidase by the method of Hamlin and Arguilla (1974), and unlabeled hormone were added and the incubation continued for 45 minutes at 20°C. Medium was then removed, cells taken off mechanically in 1.3 ml buffered saline, centrifuged in small plastic tubes, and the cell pellet counted. Maximal dilution of specific binding was achieved with 25- to 50-fold concentrations of native insulin; the counts remaining, termed nonspecific binding, comprised 39±4% of total ^{125}I-insulin binding. This nonspecific ^{125}I-

---
*Division of Genetics, Endocrinology, and Metabolism; Department of Pediatrics; University of Florida College of Medicine at Gainesville. This work was carried out while ALR was supported by a Faculty Development Award from the University of Florida.

insulin binding was 80%-90% complete at one-minute incubation.
Glucagon, prostaglandin E_1, and A and B chains of insulin did not
affect binding up to levels of 1μM. Specific binding was half-
maximal at 20 minutes, maximal at 45 minutes, and stable to 180
minute incubation. Spent medium was 90% effective with fresh CF,
indicating little insulin degradation during this incubation period.

All cell lines demonstrated 1.1%-3.6% specific binding per
10^7 cells (800-2200 molecules ^{125}I-insulin per cell) at 1 nM ^{125}I-
insulin (150 μU/ml). Increasing concentrations of ^{125}I-insulin
above 1 nM produced steeper saturation curves than could be
achieved with native insulin (Tables 1 and 2). Half saturation
with labeled hormone was reached at 2.5-7.5 nM, saturation at 10-
20 nM ^{125}I-insulin (4600-14,500 molecules ^{125}I-insulin per cell).
Genetic variation among cell strains was demonstrated by distinct
and reproducible patterns of binding throughout the saturation
curve from .05 to 30 nM ^{125}I-insulin.

Age variation was noted as a positive correlation between nonspecific binding at 1 nM ^{125}I-insulin and donor age (r=.7451, p<.01);
one progeria strain had quite high nonspecific binding for age.
Specific binding also increased significantly with donor age (r=
.5190, p<.05) with no significant differences between normal and
pathologic strains. The concentration of unlabeled insulin required to produce 50% inhibition of specific binding varied from
one to 4.5 times the concentration of ^{125}I-insulin among the nondiabetic strains, correlating positively with donor age (r=.9364,
p<.001).

Our findings in progeria have justified the expectation that
abnormality in the surface membrane insulin receptor might parallel the known defect in the surface membrane immune receptors of
the HL-A type (Singal and Goldstein, 1972). It could be postulated
that the insulin receptor undergoes alteration in its genetic expression during aging which is an underlying factor in the expression of some forms of diabetes. The greater sensitivity of young
donors' cells to competition by native insulin suggests that the
functional alteration with aging is expressed in this assay as de-
creasing negative cooperativity (DeMeyts, Roth, Neville, Gavin,
and Lesniak, 1973; DeMeyts and Roth, 1975). However, competition
curves using both lower and higher concentrations of radioiodinated
insulin indicate that the absolute concentration of insulin is not
the critical factor but rather that the ratio of labeled to native
hormone seen at 1 nM persists. This would imply that the receptor
change with aging is an increase in receptor affinity for iodoin-
sulin relative to native hormone.

Table 1. MOLECULES INSULIN BOUND PER CELL AT CONCENTRATIONS OF ^{125}I-INSULIN OF .05, .1, .25, .5, .75, AND 1.0 nM AND TOTAL INSULIN (^{125}I-INSULIN 1 nM PLUS NATIVE HORMONE) OF 2.0, 3.5, 6, 11, AND 26 nM.*

Donor age	nM ^{125}I-insulin						nM total insulin (with 1.0 nM ^{125}I-insulin)				
	.05	.1	.25	.5	.75	1.0	2.0	3.5	6	11	26
Normals: 3 mos.	120 (10)	155 (25)	320 (88)	729 (90)	749 (213)	1494 (241)	1621 (135)	1743 (38)	1152 (50)	4092 (60)	6552 (180)
10 yrs	121 (14)	183 (41)	259 (43)	787 (105)	784 (150)	1053 (174)	1308 (283)	805 (180)	900 (154)	1078 (420)	4888 (315)
22 yrs.	215 (20)	217 (55)	548 (87)	972 (137)	1602 (125)	1572 (169)	1788 (129)	2604 (235)	3132 (331)	5676 (950)	2964 (1020)
26 yrs.	591 (30)	161 (21)	395 (20)	552 (110)	1197 (167)	1149 (105)	1488 (86)	2226 (156)	2628 (694)	3762 (1023)	4329 (478)
36 yrs.	209 (27)	357 (39)	738 (108)	1344 (326)	1895 (121)	2250 (117)	3372 (98)	3066 (210)	2484 (180)	2178 (528)	9048 (936)
50 yrs.	441 (68)	179 (18)	561 (200)	1041 (280)	1053 (226)	1389 (166)	2124 (132)	3045 (515)	3492 (342)	3564 (1809)	6552 (1887)
70 yrs	173 (19)	238 (36)	779 (60)	996 (222)	1305 (192)	1898 (138)	1992 (274)	2415 (453)	2628 (444)	4664 (2124)	8112 (1764)
Progeria: 2 yrs.	424 (1)	129 (0)	219 (45)	540 (12)	743 (209)	750 (66)	887 (90)	2079 (408)	1895 (192)	2812 (223)	8211 (267)
9 yrs.	79 (11)	128 (14)	341 (30)	450 (57)	738 (71)	946 (87)	1704 (724)	2079 (478)	3348 (648)	3828 (1122)	6864 (1560)
Rothmund: 9 yrs.	145 (26)	136 (17)	383 (43)	927 (112)	1220 (18)	1206 (115)	1824 (239)	5733 (1800)	5202 (1200)	6732 (1537)	780 (311)
Lipo-atrophic 30 yrs.	104 (10)	186 (22)	445 (19)	588 (72)	896 (114)	819 (86)	888 (107)	672 (85)	252 (113)	585 (380)	2964 (488)
Diabetes: 15 yrs.	50 (6)	107 (18)	573 (19)	569 (37)	1751 (320)	1311 (14)	1260 (384)	1775 (742)	2088 (237)	2508 (1073)	5148 (993)

*Only those for which a complete series is available are shown. Numbers in parentheses are standard errors of mean for three or more determinations.

Table 2. SATURATION WITH ^{125}I-INSULIN OF FIBROBLASTS FROM THREE NORMAL CONTROLS AND THREE PERSONS WITH *IN VIVO* INSULIN RESISTANCE

Strain	Donor age						
Normal	22	1.0	3.0	6.5	18.5	29	nM*
		1248	2268	5188	8611	6090	M/C*
	10	1.0	5.0	13	37		nM
		1053	2043	2968	4828		M/C
	50	1.0	4.0	5.0	11	31	nM
		1389	5717	6255	14151	14536	M/C
Progeria	9	1.0	5.0	13	24		nM
		946	1831	2469	5427		M/C
Rothmund	9	1.0	3.0	7.0	13.6	30	nM
		1206	4296	6660	1320	0	M/C
Lipoatrophic diabetes	15	1.0	3.4	7.6	14.5	27	nM
		1311	5634	6201	8787	5508	M/C

*Molecules insulin bound per cell (M/C) shown for concentrations beginning at 1 nM.

REFERENCES

Blinstrub, R.S., Lehman, R., and Steinberg, T.H. (1964) Poikiloderma congenitale. Report of two cases. *Arch. Derm.* **89**: 659-664.

DeMeyts, P., Roth, J., Neville, D.M., Gavin, J.R. III, and Lesniak, M.A. (1973) Insulin interactions with its receptors: Experimental evidence for negative cooperativity. *Biochem. Biophys. Res. Commun.* **55**:154-161.

DeMeyts,P., and Roth, J. (1975) Insulin receptors in the cell membrane: Quantitative description of the site-site interactions. *Proc. of the 57th Annual Meeting of the Endocrine Society*, p. 51.

Flier, J.S., Kahn, C.R., Roth, J., and Bar, R.S. (1975) Antibodies that impair insulin receptor binding in an unusual diabetic syndrome with severe insulin resistance. *Science* **190**:63-65.

Hamlin, J.L. and Arguilla, E.R. (1974) Monoiodoinsulin: Preparation, purification, and characterization of a biologically active derivative substituted predominantly on Tyrosine A14. *J. Biol. Chem.* **249**:21-32.

Rosenbloom, A.L. and DeBusk, F.L. (1971) Progeria of Hutchinson-

        Gilford: A caricature of aging. *Amer. Heart J.* 82:287-289.
Singal, D.P. and Goldstein, S. (1972) Absence of detectable HL-A
        antigens on cultured fibroblasts in progeria. *J. Clin. In-*
        vest. 52:2259-2263.

DISCUSSION FOLLOWING DR. ROSENBLOOM'S TALK

Dr. Hechter
        I think this is the first hint we have that nonspecific bind-
ing may have physiological significance, at least in clinical conditions, and it raises a very interesting proposition. We have
been looking, because we are committed by our prejudice to look,
for only certain kinds of binding sites, and these we characterize
as receptors and, therefore, interesting. Other things are recognized, and we say they are not interesting. I think in a very
strange way you have called our attention to the fact that there
may be hidden in this mess elements of the greatest significance
with respect to aging and with respect to disease, and so I would
like to thank you very much.

Dr. Rosenbloom
        Thank you.

Dr. Forte
        Did you explain your binding assay; was this binding of insulin
to the cells or was it binding to the cell membranes after solubilization?

Dr. Rosenbloom
        This assay is done in the 100-millimeter petri dish with any-
where from a million and a half to four or five million cells, depending on how many there are at confluence, which is an individual
characteristic of the cell strain. Incubation is completed at room
temperature with the insulin-containing medium overlying the intact
monolayer. Using a siliconized rubber policeman the cells are
scraped off in the PBS, aspirated in a siliconized pipette, trans-
ferred to a microcentrifuge tube, spun down, supernatant removed,
and the tip clipped off and counted.

SUBJECT INDEX

Printed in the United States
by Baker & Taylor Publisher Services

Printed in the United States
by Baker & Taylor Publisher Services